CHURCHILL'S

House Surgeon's Survival Guide

CHURCHILL'S

House Surgeon's Survival Guide

Second Edition

R. HENRY K. GOMPERTZ MS FRCS
Consultant Surgeon, Burton Hospitals
NHS Trust, Burton–on–Trent, UK

MICHAEL RHODES MA(Cantab) BMBCh(Oxon) MD FRCS
Consultant Surgeon, Norfolk and Norwich Hospital
Norwich, UK

GRAEME J. POSTON MB MS FRCS(Ed) FRCS(Eng)
Consultant Surgeon, Royal Liverpool University Hospital
Liverpool, UK

Second Edition revised by

Bart Decadt MD FRCS
Specialist Registrar, Hope Hospital, Manchester, UK

Jon Armitage MBChB
Senior House Officer in Surgery, Leeds General Infirmary,
Leeds, UK

CHURCHILL
LIVINGSTONE

EDINBURGH LONDON NEW YORK PHILADELPHIA ST LOUIS SYDNEY
TORONTO 2000

CHURCHILL LIVINGSTONE
An imprint of Harcourt Publishers Limited

© Longman Group UK Limited 1992
© Harcourt Publishers Limited 2000

The right of R Henry Gompertz, Michael Rhodes and
Graeme J Poston to be identified as authors of this work has
been asserted by them in accordance with the Copyright,
Designs and Patents Act 1988

First edition 1992
Second edition 2000

ISBN 0443 06223 4

International Student Edition
ISBN 0443 06222 6

British Library Cataloguing in Publication Data
A catalogue record for this book is available from the British
Library

Library of Congress Cataloging in Publication Data
A catalog record for this book is available from the Library of
Congress

Note
Medical knowledge is constantly changing. As new
information becomes available, changes in treatment,
procedures, equipment and the use of drugs become
necessary. The authors and the publishers have, as far as it is
possible, taken care to ensure that the information given in
this text is accurate and up-to-date. However, readers are
strongly advised to confirm that the information, especially
with regard to drug usage, complies with the latest legislation
and standards of practice.

The
publisher's
policy is to use
**paper manufactured
from sustainable forests**

Printed in China

Following the success of the first edition of the House Surgeon's Survival Guide, we are very grateful to Harcourt Publishers to be invited to produce a second edition.

In the six years since the first edition much has changed. Surgery has become more specialised and the educational component of the pre-registration year more structurally defined. On-call commitments have been reduced by law and therefore hands-on experience in turn is diminished.

We hope that this second edition will continue to offer guidance, advice and support during this often difficult transition from student to practising doctor.

R. H. K. G.   B. D.
Burton on Trent   Manchester

M. R.   J. A.
Norwich   Leeds

G. J. P.
Liverpool

PREFACE TO FIRST EDITION

It's 3 am in the morning, your first night on call as a House Surgeon and the phone rings. 'Hello, is that Dr Newboy? Mrs Diehard is in a lot of pain – can you sort her out?' What next? Nobody ever gave us a lecture about this, you think. A quick fumble through the pages of your chosen textbook reveals that it too has nothing to offer. You stumble across from the doctors' residence, mind wandering, pulse racing and finally resolve to appear cool, calm and in control when you arrive on the ward. Wouldn't it be nice if someone, somewhere had written something to help you in such situations.

The House Surgeon's Survival Guide is just such a book. Its four sections guide the reader through the realities of life as a Surgical House Officer. Life on the wards, routine admissions, emergency admissions, the theatre list and personal life are all covered with helpful hints, tables and algorithms to guide you through the day.

It is not an exhaustive textbook or another short notes book which supplements pre-finals cramming. If you want to make a fool of yourself on a ward round by knowing everything there is to know about von Willebrand's disease, then you must look elsewhere. If, however, you want to *survive* surgery, then this book is for you. Written by three medics who are still surviving surgery as a Lecturer, Career Registrar and Consultant, it aims to provide practical guidelines for the formative few months of your surgical house job, the success of which can significantly determine your subsequent career prospects. If you are unsure how to place a urinary catheter or investigate postoperative chest pain – it's in here. If you wonder about the management of diabetes in the surgical patient or how to prepare somebody for a thyroidectomy, read on. Even if you just want to know how to persuade the biochemist to do a difficult out-of-hours investigation, this book will help you.

Also, this book is intended to be of use to final year medical students as they begin their 'shadow' attachments to Surgical House Officers in the months before their finals.

We hope our readers do *survive* surgery and, with the aid of this book, enjoy their time in surgery.

R.H.K.G.
Newcastle 1992

M.R.
Bristol 1992

G.J.P.
Liverpool 1992

This book is drawn from our cumulative experience with significant contributions and advice from others, most notably newly qualified House Surgeons who were crying out for a vade mecum such as this. We would particularly like to thank Austin Leach, Consultant Anaesthetist, Royal Liverpool Hospital, for his contributions to the anaesthesia sections, and Andy James, Consultant and Senior Lecturer in Endocrinology at the RVI in Newcastle, and Peter Reid, Consultant Cardiologist, Countess of Chester Hospital in Chester, for their help and advice on the sections regarding the medical management of the surgical patient.

We are indebted to the help and support of Lucy Gardner and Jim Killgore at Churchill Livingstone during the evolution and fruition of this project, and Dr Amr Radwan for offering suggestions at proof stage.

Finally we thank our wives Jill, Jenny and June for their patience and fortitude, not only through this project but for the many moves, long weekends on call and financial hardships endured because of our surgical ambitions. This book is dedicated to them.

ABBREVIATIONS

ABG	arterial blood gases
ACE	angiotensin converting enzyme
AIDS	acquired immunodeficiency syndrome
APTT	activated partial thromboplastin time
AXR	abdominal X-ray
b.d.	twice daily
bpm	beats per minute
CABG	coronary artery bypass graft
CBD	common bile duct
CCF	congestive cardiac failure
CNS	central nervous system
COPD	chronic obstructive pulmonary disease
CPR	cardiopulmonary resuscitation
CSF	cerebrospinal fluid
CSU	catheter specimen of urine
CT	computerized tomography
CVA	cerebro–vascular accident
CVP	central venous pressure
CVS	cardiovascular system
CXR	chest X-ray
DIC	disseminated intravascular coagulation
DPL	diagnostic peritoneal lavage
DU	duodenal ulcer
DVT	deep venous thrombosis
ECG	electrocardiogram
EEG	electroencephalogram
EMG	electromyography
ERCP	endoscopic retrograde cholangiopancreatography
ESR	erythrocyte sedimentation rate
ET	endotracheal
EUA	examination under anaesthetic
FBC	full blood count
FEV_1	forced expiratory volume in 1 second
FFP	fresh frozen plasma
FNAB	fine needle aspiration biopsy
FVC	forced vital capacity
G&S/XM	group & save/cross match
GA	general anaesthesia
GKI	glucose/potassium/insulin
GTN	glyceryl trinitrate
GU	gastric ulcer
Hb	haemoglobin
HBV	hepatitis B virus
HIV	human immunodeficiency virus
HRT	hormone replacement therapy
IBD	inflammatory bowel disease
IDDM	insulin-dependent diabetes mellitus

IHD	ischaemic heart disease
i.m.	intramuscularly
INR	international normalized ratio
i.v.	intravenously
IVC	inferior vena cava
IVU	intravenous urogram
JVP	jugular venous pressure
KCCT	koalin cephalin clotting time
LFT	liver function test
LIF	left iliac fossa
LUQ	left upper quandrant
mane	in the morning
MCHC	mean corpuscular haemoglobin concentration
MC&S	microscopy, culture and sensitivity
MCV	mean corpuscular volume
mg	milligram
μg	microgram
MI	myocardial infarction
MIBG	met-iodo benzol guanidine
MLSO	medical laboratory scientific officer
MSSU	midstream specimen of urine
MSU	midstream urine
NG	nasogastric
NIDDM	non-insulin dependent diabetes mellitus
NSAID	non-steroidal anti-inflammatory drugs
nocte	at night
o.d.	once daily
OCP	oral contraceptive pill
PCV	packed cell volume
PE	pulmonary embolism
p.o.	oral
p.r.	per rectum
prn	as required
PSA	prostate specific antigen
PTC	percutaneous transhepatic cholangiogram
PTH	parathyroid hormone
PVD	peripheral vascular disease
q.d.s.	four times daily
RCC	red cell count
RIF	right iliac fossa
RUQ	right upper quadrant
SCBU	special care baby unit
SHO	senior house officer
SOBOE	shortness of breath on exertion
SPR	specialist registrar
TB	tuberculosis
TBG	thyroid binding globulin
TIA	transient ischaemic attack
t.d.s.	three times daily
TPN	total parenteral nutrition
TSH	thyroid stimulating hormone

TURP	transurethral resection of the prostate
U	unit
U & E	urea and electrolytes
URTI	upper respiratory tract infection
USS	ultrasound scan
UTI	urinary tract infection
VF	ventricular fibrillation
VT	ventricular tachycardia
WBC	white blood count
WCC	white cell count

Introduction

Congratulations! Now you are a doctor and about to start your Surgical House Job. Will you survive? For many people in this situation the answer is an unqualified 'yes', but there are many others for whom the answer is, 'I hope so'. The difficulties of each post will be different. A great deal depends on the personal resources of the individual House Surgeon. A great deal more depends on the particular post and hospital. Teaching hospital jobs tend to have a smaller throughput of patients (but not always) and these patients tend to be more complicated and require more investigations and more prolonged management. District general hospital jobs are often very busy in terms of throughput but are more relaxed. This book aims to make it easier for you to handle any situation and to emerge from the Surgical House Job intact, enthused and ready for your next challenge. Good luck!

SURVIVING THE HOUSE SURGEON'S DAY

Most House Surgeons will start the day with a ward round. You will not normally be expected to do this on your own, and there may be a set timetable for which days have Consultant ward rounds and which are led by either the SPR or SHO.

Ward rounds should be enjoyable! As the doctor with the most ward contact, you should direct the ward round, leading the team from patient to patient giving an update on condition and test results as you go. Even the most fearsome consultants are usually consistent; if for some reason he likes to know daily stool volumes, there's little point complaining – have the results ready and watch his joy as he thinks he's converted his young house officer to his ways!! (Just think of the reference.)

At the end of the round you will normally be left to get on with a list of jobs (investigations, referrals, etc.) in your own time. It's very tempting to now disappear off to the mess for a coffee but you will find that jobs don't just go away so organize the list into the following categories:

1. Things to be done straightaway.
2. Things to be done that day.
3. Things to be done sometime, but which can wait.

Things to be done straightaway

Emergencies, either on the ward or in A & E, make up the first category. The order of priority with these patients is:

- Resuscitation where necessary: call for help (crash team, etc.) and start resuscitation
- **A**irway (with cervical spine control in trauma)
- **B**reathing: ventilation and oxygenation
- **C**irculation:
  – two large-calibre peripheral intravenous lines in trauma
  – send blood tests now (cross-matching, U & E, clotting, gases, FBC and glucose)
- **D**isability (neurological evaluation, see page 126) and **D**rugs.

This **ABCD** logical, sequential assessment and treatment can be applied as a starting management in all emergencies, including polytrauma, cardiac arrest, head injury, respiratory arrest, etc. Using this sequence will help you not to omit essential steps in each emergency (e.g. it makes little sense to do a neurological assessment in a postoperatively confused patient before assessing airway, breathing and circulation).

- Order emergency investigations (ECG, CXR, CT, etc.).
- Alert other personnel where appropriate (theatre, anaesthetist, surgeon, etc.).

For emergency admissions not so ill as to require the same degree of haste in their management, there are still some things more important than others. To the House Surgeon the most important thing often seems to be that they know exactly what is going on with the patient; funnily enough this can, occasionally, be the last thing that matters. An emergency admission usually will already have been seen by someone more senior and a plan of action made. Your first priority is to implement that plan. Note-keeping and clerking are important, but can wait. A patient's operation will be deferred because of lack of investigations, but rarely because the House Surgeon has not taken a full history.

Things to be done that day

Bloods Several administrative tasks must be done. Bloods must be sent off and investigations requested, first thing in the morning, so that they can be attended to that day. Speed the process up as follows:

- Blood bottles should not be prelabelled (*don't put the wrong blood into the wrong bottle!*)

- Make out the blood forms in advance
- Have the appropriate envelopes ready.

If you have help with blood-taking from medical students or phlebotomists, delegate the less important bloods to them. There is nothing more frustrating than finding that a medical student has failed to get a blood and not told you about it, and as a result the patient has had his/her operation deferred.

The most important investigations are those that are likely to be acted upon, i.e. preoperative ones and those for patients who are ill. Routine postoperative bloods must be taken, but have a lower priority; if you are really busy, these can be deferred.

Radiology   Requests should be discussed with the radiology department if they are at all urgent or complicated. This is the only way to make sure you get the test you want when you want it.

Consultations   These must be arranged – letters requesting consultation should, wherever possible, be hand delivered (then you *know* they have been received).

Discharge letters/prescriptions   must be written so that the patient can be discharged (and the next one admitted). If possible, try to prepare discharge prescriptions in advance of the ward round as these can take several hours for the pharmacy to produce.

Clerking of routine patients   comes further down the list of priorities, and in any case, these patients usually come in after mid-morning so the work from the morning's ward round should be out of the way. When patients come in:

- Read the notes and find out:
  – what they have been admitted for
  – what investigations need to be done.

  The latter are often written in the last outpatient appointment or in the last letter from the GP. Sometimes there will be a definite management plan written out for you to follow; at other times you will have to deduce it.

- Take bloods and send them off for appropriate investigations
- Arrange other tests.

You can talk to and examine the patient any time.

Eating and drinking   Despite what you may think, it is rare for you to be too busy to grab a drink and something to eat. You will probably find that 10 min sat eating a sandwich or bar of chocolate will allow you to work more quickly later on.

Things to be done sometime, but which can wait

- Record-keeping (audit)

- Routine note-keeping
- Eating and sleeping.

Record-keeping Note-keeping is a vital part of the House Surgeon's work and in many cases you will be expected to keep notes on behalf of other people – in other words, for consultations and visits by other members of staff. Although it is ideal if everybody makes their own notes, in real life this often fails to happen and it therefore falls to the House Surgeon to make good the shortfall. The following notes are essential.

Clerking on admission

- The paper that you write on should be properly fixed into the notes.
- Every page must be headed with the patient's name and hospital (record) number.
- The date and time of entry should be noted on every occasion.
- Each clerking should be organized in the usual way:
  - Presenting complaint
  - History
  - Examination
  - Differential diagnosis
  - Investigations
  - Plan.

Leave room when you write in the planned investigations to make a note of the results when they come back.

Remember

An investigation has not been done until the results are in the notes.

Progress After the initial admission, investigations and plan have been noted, it is best if some sort of note is made every day, although for long-stay patients every 2 or 3 days may be reasonable, provided nothing is happening.

New events Complications, consultations, investigations, new treatments, visits to the theatre and returns to the ward from recovery all must be recorded in the notes.

Every time you are called to see a patient, you should make a comment in the notes. You should be aware that if you are bleeped by a nurse, who says, 'Oh by the way, I thought I would just tell you about such and such about so and so', they will almost certainly have written in the nursing kardex 'doctor informed', whereupon any subsequent problem is *your* problem.

Discharge A summary should be made in the notes on the discharge of the patient, including:

- Date of discharge

- outpatient follow-up planned
- investigations that have been organized as an outpatient
- any further specific treatment or arrangement for readmission.

Patients should leave with some form of discharge letter in their hand, and ideally they should have an outpatient appointment as well, rather than this being sent by post.

Other forms of note-keeping

- Keeping a list of deaths and complications for the audit meeting.
- Keeping careful notes of what has been explained to patients (e.g. for patients with a diagnosis of malignant disease – Do they know? Do their relatives know?).
- Any sign of complaint.
- If patients have been given special instructions or warned particularly of specific complications.
- Important interviews: 'Mr Bloggs, discussed the problem with Mrs Smith and her relatives…'

Remember

The most common reason for failure to defend medical staff successfully in legal cases is poor note-keeping.

SECTION 1

Surviving on the wards

1

Clerking elective admissions

CLERKING TECHNIQUE

The spectrum of patients admitted as 'elective' is broad. They range from the routine admission of fit patients for relatively minor procedures (e.g. veins, hernias) to urgent admissions from clinic who may be as sick as emergency admissions through A & E. Between these extremes are those patients with minor surgical problems but major intercurrent illnesses. In this chapter the presenting problem itself will be dealt with. Patients with acute problems admitted as 'elective' can be managed using the advice in the emergency section of this book (page 133). Advice on intercurrent medical problems is also given in a separate chapter (page 47).

Here you will find systems for focusing attention on the problem in hand. However, as the House Surgeon you will also be expected to have looked at the patient in a broader and more systematic way. The assessment of the surgical patient aims to confirm and clarify the diagnosis, detect and deal with unsuspected intercurrent illness, and assess fitness for anaesthesia. This book does not aim to be an exhaustive textbook of surgery, and this chapter is not intended to cover the most basic points of history-taking and examination. The purpose is rather to improve and rationalize technique and to maximize efficiency.

The end result of successful clerking should be organized case notes, a definite management plan, a crisp presentation on formal ward rounds and no important points overlooked.

HISTORY

Surgical history-taking should not usually take more than 5 min and can overlap with examination:

- The history should start with the patient's *name, age* and *occupation*.
- Questions to discover the *presenting problem* and *associated symptoms* should be asked and you should make a general systematic enquiry about *diet* and *gastrointestinal, urinary, respiratory, cardiac* and *neurological* problems.
- An accurate *drug* and *allergy* history is essential together with *past medical history*.
- *Social history* should include use of recreational drugs, including nicotine and alcohol. *Sexual* practices should be tactfully enquired about – if you don't ask you may miss important information; the degree of detail may depend on initial findings and the presenting complaint.

EXAMINATION

The physical examination should be both general and specific and take about 10 min. A nurse or colleague should always be asked to act as chaperone when examining patients of the opposite sex.

General features   Include fitness, nutritional status and 'biological age'. Look for **j**aundice, **a**naemia, **c**lubbing, **c**yanosis, **o**edemata and **l**ymphadenopathy (remember JACCOL), together with examination of the hands, eyes, mouth, neck and breasts in every case.

Systemic features   Do a general 'overview' examination:

- Cardiovascular system
- Respiratory system
- Abdomen
- Neurological system.

An 'overview' examination of the abdomen and the main systems is done routinely for anaesthetic assessment and to detect unsuspected concurrent disease.

Specific examination   If relevant to the presenting complaint, this must be detailed. Findings, both positive and negative, must be carefully documented with measurements if appropriate (e.g. size of lump).

> **Remember**
>
> Four things that are commonly omitted:
>
> - Record blood pressure, temperature and pulse; if necessary, measure them yourself.
> - Always do a rectal examination (where physically possible).
> - If clinically indicated, do examine the female breast.
> - Make sure that a sample has been sent for urinalysis.

The basic method outlined in Table 1.1 can be made most efficient by a systematic approach to clerking, particularly in the timing of investigations. Checking for tests already arranged, or suggested, by the outpatient doctor will prevent you from duplicating work or missing out something important. The best and worst clerking techniques are summarized in Table 1.2.

PLAN OF ACTION

- Skim through the notes looking specifically for recent admissions and outpatient/discharge letters. Taking the notes, walk to the patient's bedside. If they are not in bed or ready to be examined, use this time to fill in their blood forms or book relevant tests.

Table 1.1
Clerking checklist

History
Basics (name, age, occupation)
Presenting problem (duration, progression, predisposition, secondary effects)
Previous medical history (serious illnesses, operations)
Family history
Social history (marital status, children, drugs, allergies, alcohol, tobacco)
Systematic enquiry (usually tailored to presenting complaint)

Examination
General impression (fitness for age, in pain/comfortable, ill)
Hands (clubbing, Dupuytren's, nails, skin colour, perfusion, pulse)
Eyes (pallor, jaundice, fundi, xanthelasmata)
Mouth (hydration, hygiene, dentition)
Neck (nodes, especially supraclavicular fossa)
Breast (*always* in the female, also chest wall, e.g. spider naevi)
Abdomen (tone/tenderness, liver, spleen, kidneys, other lumps, groin, PR)
Blood pressure
Urinalysis

Investigations
FBC, ESR
U & E, LFTs
CXR
ECG
Specific investigations

- Introduce yourself, check the patient's name and write down their age and occupation.
- Ask what the problem is. After one or two sentences of the answer say, 'Let's have a look then'. As the patient undresses keep asking relevant questions.
- Examine the relevant part and at the same time ask questions relevant to the primary problem, secondary effects, underlying causes and general features.
- Do a general 'overview' examination (respiratory, cardiovascular, neurological, etc.) whilst asking 'overview' questions.
- Look at the last note before admission. What special instructions are given?

> **Table 1.2**
> **Methods of information gathering**
>
> | **Traditional method** | |
> | --- | --- |
> | Technique | Result |
> | | |
> | *History* | |
> | History of everything | |
> | – List of negatives | Bores clinician to death |
> | – All trees no wood | Patient dies of neglect |
> | | |
> | *Examination* | |
> | Examine everything | |
> | – Takes a week | May be technical assault |
> | – Signs masked by boredom | Patient sues doctor |
> | | |
> | *Investigations* | |
> | Every known test | |
> | – High cost/low yield | Patient dies of anaemia |
> | – Irrelevant abnormalities | Relatives sue doctor |
>
> *End up wondering what is wrong and where to go next – a headless chicken*
>
> | **Problem-solving method** | |
> | --- | --- |
> | Technique | Result |
> | | |
> | *History* | |
> | Ask the right question | |
> | – 'What is the matter?' | Discover relevant facts |
> | – Specific questions | Identify area of problem |
> | | |
> | *Examination* | |
> | Look in the right place | |
> | – 'Let's have a look' | Elicit relevant signs |
> | – Specific signs | Close in on problem |
> | | |
> | *Investigations* | |
> | Do the right test | |
> | – 'One or two tests' | First- and second-line tests |
> | – Specific investigations | The detailed problem |
>
> *End up with clear diagnosis and plan – a problem solved*

– Does the patient need specific investigations or blood tests? Do these now. Don't do one blood test after another
– Are any special tests booked or do any need booking? Arrange these now

– Does the patient need any specific preparation (e.g. bowel prep or DVT prophylaxis)? Write these up along with their regular medication
– Is the patient to be booked for theatre? If so, consent and include on list.
• Write in the notes: history, examination, investigations and plan of action.

MALIGNANT DISEASE

The patient admitted for investigation or management of possible malignant disease must be clerked with special care because the House Surgeon may be the only person to do a *thorough examination of all parts*. Even if the patient has been seen very recently before admission, it is important to go over everything again because symptoms and signs change as the disease progresses. A patient who is on the ward for more than a few days during the course of investigation should be re-examined thoroughly because new signs may have appeared.

The responsibility of the doctor to the *whole* patient is probably greater for those with malignant disease than with almost any other illness. In addition to the main problem with which the patient has presented or for which they are being investigated (e.g. jaundice, weight loss, abdominal mass, etc.), there may be *many other symptoms* that need investigation and treatment. Typical symptoms include nausea and vomiting (other than where due to specific problems such as bowel obstruction), pain, general malaise, etc. *Psychological and spiritual support* may be required and contact should be made with suitable persons to deal with these matters. Honesty in discussing diagnosis and prognosis is required but avoid brutal honesty – leave the patient some hope (see talking to patients and relative, page 240). Discuss with your consultant if the patient is for active resuscitation or not. The family should be informed about this medical decision. *Write the consultant's decision and 'discussed with family' in the notes*. This will save a lot of trouble for the patient, the family and the caring team in case the patient arrests.

Where *terminal care* may be required, either at home or in an appropriate institution, *start making arrangements as soon as possible*. Dying on an acute ward is noisy and lacks privacy and the ward staff, both medical and nursing, rarely have the skills in caring for the terminally ill that can be found in specialized services.

Checklists for clerking patients with the common malignancies found on surgical wards are given in Tables 1.3–1.6.

Table 1.3
Checklist for clerking patient with colonic cancer (Left=left-sided, Right=right-sided)

		Primary tumour	Secondary spread	General effects
Symptoms	Left:	Change of bowel habit (constipation or diarrhoea) Rectal bleeding Obstruction Tenesmus	RUQ mass/ pain (liver) Abdominal swelling Weight loss	Weight loss Weakness
	Right:	Change of bowel habit (diarrhoea) RIF mass Pain	As above	As above
Signs	Left:	Palpable tumour (LIF or PR) Signs of obstruction Blood on PR glove Anaemia	Hepatomegaly (knobbly) Ascites Jaundice Supraclavicular node	Loose clothes Wasting
	Right:	RIF mass Normocytic anaemia	As above	As above
Tests		FBC Faecal occult blood Sigmoidoscopy USS (liver) Laparoscopy and laparoscopic USS	U & E, LFTs Ascitic tap Barium enema and/or colonoscopy CT scan (rarely)	

Left-sided lesions tend to present early because the bowel is narrow and the contents solid. Late presentation with metastatic disease occurs but is less common by far than in right-sided disease.
Right-sided lesions obstruct late with extracolonic spread because the bowel diameter is wide and the contents fluid.

Table 1.4
Checklist for clerking patient with breast cancer

	Primary tumour	Secondary spread	General effects
Symptoms	Lump in breast Mastalgia (breast pain) (rarely) Nipple discharge (bloody)	Lump in axilla Abdominal swelling (ascites) RUQ mass/pain (liver) Cough/shortness of breath Headaches/neurological problems	Weight loss
Signs	Lump in breast Bloody nipple discharge Normocytic anaemia Skin changes (puckering, peau d'orange, discoloration, ulceration)	Axillary lymphadenopathy Ascites Pleural effusion Hepatomegaly (knobbly) Neurological signs Bone pain	Loose clothes, wasting
Tests	Fine needle cytology Mammogram USS (breast) Open biopsy/lumpectomy	FBC, U & E, LFTs Bone scan/skeletal survey USS (liver) Ascitic tap/CT scans	

Table 1.5
Checklist for clerking patient with gastric cancer

	Primary tumour	Secondary spread	General effects
Symptoms	Nausea/vomiting Haematemesis/melaena Dysphagia Weight loss Epigastric tenderness	RUQ mass/pain (liver) Abdominal swelling (ascites)	Weight loss
Signs	Epigastric mass Anaemia Succussion splash (pyloric obstruction)	Hepatomegaly (knobbly) Ascites Jaundice Supraclavicular node Rectal mass (transcoelomic)	Loose clothes, wasting
Tests	FBC Faecal occult blood Barium meal Endoscopy	U & E, LFTs Ascitic tap USS (liver) CT scan Laparoscopy and laparoscopic USS	

In the UK, gastric cancer often presents late with symptoms and signs both from the primary tumour and secondary spread.

Table 1.6
Checklist for clerking patient with pancreatic cancer

	Primary tumour	Secondary spread	General effects
Symptoms	Jaundice Epigastric pain Gastric outflow obstruction	RUQ mass/pain (liver) Abdominal swelling (ascites)	Weight loss
Signs	Jaundice Epigastric mass Palpable gallbladder Anaemia	Hepatomegaly (knobbly) Ascites Supraclavicular node	Loose clothes, wasting
Tests	LFTs USS (needle biopsy) ERCP (brush cytology) PTC (brush cytology) CT (needle biopsy)	FBC, U & E Ascitic tap USS (liver) Laparoscopy and laparoscopic USS	

EXAMINATION OF A LUMP

Look (7 × S)

- **S**ite, position
- **S**ize: measure in two directions and thickness where possible
- **S**hape
- **S**urface: seek associated scars, sinuses, atrophy, and loss of hair
- **S**urrounding: check for regional lymphadenopathy
- **S**kin: colour at rest and with pressure
- **S**hine a light: translucency.

Feel (3 × T)

- **T**enderness
- **T**emperature
- **T**exture: smooth, rough or bosselated?
  hard, rubbery, spongy or soft?
- Press on it: pulsatile/expansile?
  compressible/reducible?
  cough impulse?
  fluid thrill?
- Remember to feel its edge and all around it
  Discrete or ill defined?
  Can you get above/below/beside it?
  Is it causing a functional deficit, circulatory, motor or neurological?
  Is there regional/general lymphadenopathy or hepatosplenomegaly?

Move

- Does the lump move spontaneously or with respiration?
- Does the skin move over the lump? Tethered?
- Does the lump move over underlying structures? Which directions?
- Repeat movements with the patient tensing underlying muscles.

Listen

- Bruit
- Bowel sounds.

Investigate

- X-ray
  - Calcification
  - Definition of other structures
  - Contrast studies (including displacement or invasion of nearby structures)

- Ultrasound
  - Internal architecture: solid or cystic, homogeneous or heterogeneous?
- Aspiration
  - Cytology: useful for any superficial lump
  - Microscopy for bacteria culture and sensitivity.

HEAD AND NECK LUMPS

The most common cause for a lump in the neck is an enlarged lymph node with the most common aetiological factors being infection and secondary tumour deposits. However, a lump may arise from any structure that may be found in that anatomical area, whether it be present normally or as a congenital anomaly. Here organ-specific lumps will be considered, but other lumps such as those arising from skin, subcutaneous tissue, fat and muscle should not be forgotten when examining the head and neck.

In order to make a diagnosis of a lump in the neck the following steps should be carried out:

1. Examination of the lump in order to answer four key questions:
   (a) Site of the swelling? (anatomical area, Fig. 1.1)
   (b) Solid or cystic?
   (c) Does it move with swallowing?
   (d) Is it single or multiple? (multiple swellings are usually lymphatic).
2. A specific history.
3. A general examination for associated signs (secondary features).
4. Special investigations.

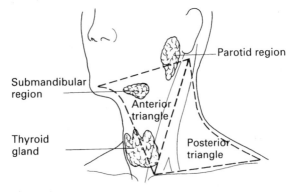

Fig. 1.1 Regions of the neck

ANTERIOR MIDLINE

Specific structures

- Thyroid
- Thyroid-associated lumps – ectopic thyroid and thyroglossal cyst
- Parathyroids (very rarely palpable)
- True dermoid cyst.

The physical sign to elicit in this area is that of moving on swallowing:

- All thyroid swellings ascend during swallowing, but not on protrusion of the tongue. If a lump moves up both on swallowing and protrusion of the tongue, it must be attached to the hyoid bone, and be a thyroglossal cyst.
- Thyroglossal swellings move both on swallowing and protrusion of the tongue.

Testing for movement both on swallowing and tongue protrusion is easy to do badly. To detect movement on tongue protrusion, the patient should be asked to open their mouth and then to protrude the tongue. If the patient is just asked to stick out their tongue, both movements will take place simultaneously. This means that as the mouth opens the muscles suspending the thyroglossal tract relax and as the tongue protrudes they contract, and the net effect may be that there is no visible movement. To detect movement on swallowing the patient should be instructed to take a gulp of water into the mouth but not to swallow it until the mouth is closed and you are ready to observe carefully.

The same technique should be used for both inspection and palpation. Inspection should take place from the front and the side. Palpation should be done from the front and from behind the patient. Movement is felt better if the lump is gently pushed down to take up any 'slack' in the muscles, thus accentuating it.

Thyroid

Specific features

Look

- First confirm that the swelling is in the thyroid: does it ascend on swallowing?
- Observe the surface and contours of the swelling: the skin may be puckered if a thyroid carcinoma has infiltrated the skin.
- Try to transilluminate any superficial cystic swelling.
- Look inside the mouth for ectopic thyroid tissue at the back of the tongue and fossa.
- Is the thyroid cartilage in the centre of the neck or deviated?
- The neck veins are distended if there is a mass obstructing the thoracic outlet.

Feel

- Tenderness, shape, size, surface and consistency. A normal thyroid gland is not palpable.
- Position of the trachea.
- Is there fixation to surrounding structures?
- Are there any regional lymph nodes?
- Percuss to ascertain whether there is retrosternal extension.

Listen

- A vascular lump may have a systolic bruit (ask patient to hold breath).

Specific history

- Ask about the voice change and dysphagia, listen to speech.

Secondary features

- Eyes — exophthalmos, lid retraction, lid lag, ocular paresis (hyperthyroid)
  — loss of eyebrow (hypothyroid)
- Sympathetic — tremor, tachycardia and irregular rhythm (hyperthyroid)
  — bradycardia (hypothyroid)
- Bowels — diarrhoea (hyperthyroid)
  — constipation (hypothyroid)
- Menses — amenorrhoea (hyperthyroid)
  — menorrhagia (hypothyroid)
- Weight — decrease (hyperthyroid)
  — increase (hypothyroid)
- Sleep — little (hyperthyroid)
  — lots (hypothyroid)
- Weather — likes cold (hyperthyroid)
  — likes hot (hypothyroid)
- Skin — hot moist (hyperthyroid)
  — coarse, dry (hypothyroid).

Key investigations

- Electrolytes, FBC
- Thyroid function tests — T4, T3, TSH, TBG
- Neck ultrasound — multiple or single lesions, solid or cystic
- Isotope uptake scanning — cold (no uptake), warm (same as the rest of the gland), hot (intense uptake in area of lump with suppression of the rest of the gland)
- Fine-needle aspiration cytology — cell type (NB. Cannot always tell benign from malignant)
- CXR, thoracic inlet views — for tracheal deviation, retrosternal goitre.

Thyroglossal cyst

Look

- Position close to the midline
- Overlying skin red, hot and tender if cyst is infected
- A thyroglossal cyst is always closely related to the hyoid bone (ask patient to protrude the tongue).

Feel

- They fluctuate if not too tense.

Move

- They are tethered by the remnant of the thyroglossal duct, so they can be moved sideways, but not up and down.

Dermoid cyst

- Check nodes
- Transilluminate (usually won't, murky contents).

Parathyroids

Specific features

- Rarely palpable. If so may move with thyroid (especially upper)
- Check nodes.

Secondary symptoms and signs

- Features of hypercalcaemia (stones, bones, abdominal groans)
  - stones
  - abdominal pain (non-specific or specific, e.g. pancreatitis)
  - bone pain
  - psychiatric problems.

Special investigations

- Calcium (total and ionized)
- Parathyroid hormone (abnormal if detectable with high calcium).

ANTERIOR TRIANGLE

Specific swellings

- Branchial cyst
- Carotid body tumour
- Carotid aneurysm.

Specific features

- Obviously, the latter two pulsate, whereas the former does not

- Massage of the carotid body tumour is a bad idea
- All usually have bruits
- Branchial cysts feel like cysts.

Special investigations

- Ultrasound
- Doppler studies
- Angiography (venous phase if need be).

POSTERIOR TRIANGLE

Lymph node

SUPRACLAVICULAR FOSSA

- Innominate or subclavian aneurysms
- Lymph node (Virchov's node on the left-hand side where the thoracic duct drains).

SUBMANDIBULAR AREA

Submandibular salivary gland

Specific features

- Pain on eating
- Look inside the mouth and palpate the floor of the mouth.

Secondary features

- Lymph nodes
- Immune disorder (Sjögren's).

Special investigations

- Sialography
- Immune studies.

PAROTID AREA

Specific swellings

- Parotid gland
- External angular dermoid.

Parotid gland

Specific features

- May deform the pinna
- Asymmetry (look at both sides)
- Assess VIIth cranial nerve on both sides (ask the patient to smile and screw up eyes)
- History of pain on eating

- Skin for colour, scars, sinuses
- Look and feel inside the mouth at the area of the 2nd upper molar (the point of entry of the parotid duct) for pus, stone, lump.

Secondary features

- Regional lymphadenopathy
- Features of generalized disease (mumps, Sjögren's, rheumatoid).

Special investigations

- Plain film (calcific stone)
- Sialography
- Immune studies
- FNAB.

External angular dermoid

This is a true dermoid formed as a result of an abnormality of diffusion of the facial plates.

LYMPHADENOPATHY

A comprehensive differential diagnosis for the causes of lymphadenopathy is beyond the scope of this book. It can be localized or generalized.

Localized

1. Local infection
2. Metastatic tumour
3. Lymphoma.

Generalized

1. Infection (e.g. EBV, CMV, toxoplasma, TB)
2. Leukaemia
3. Lymphoma
4. Systemic inflammatory disease (e.g. RA, SLE).

The examinations you will be expected to have done are:

- History
- Examination of a lump (see p. 19)
- General examination (with the main causes of enlargement in your mind)
  including examination of the area that the nodes drain, liver and spleen examination
- Investigations
  - FBC and viral studies
  - FNAB or better an excision biopsy (contact the pathology department beforehand and ask how they want the specimen).

25

BREAST PROBLEMS

There are many diseases that may affect the breast and many ways for these to present. For practical purposes, however, there are four common presentations:

1. A lump (painful or painless)
2. Pain
3. Nipple discharge/change
4. Changes in breast size.

Lump

There are three common lumps:

- Fibroadenoma – usual age 15–35 years
- Cyst – usual age 35–45 years
- Cancer – usual age 45+ years.

Less common lumps include:

- Giant fibroadenoma
- Fat necrosis – history of trauma
- Abscess – infected cyst, trauma, lactation
- Rare tumours – sarcoma, metastasis, etc.
- Other tissues nearby – skin, fat, muscle, bone, cartilage.

Pain

Pain ('mastalgia') is common and usually means benign disease:

- Cyclical
- Associated with periods (worst just before)
- Generally lumpy breasts, often asymmetrical
- Pain and tenderness commonest in the axillary tail.

Localized pain may have a trigger point:

- Not cycle related
- Well localized
- Worse in cold weather
- Sometimes trauma related
- Due to localized mammary dysplasia.

Rarer causes include:

- Pregnancy – commonly sore, rarely sent to surgeon
- Cancer – even with no palpable lump
- Tietz's disease – costochondritis
- Mondor's disease – venous thrombosis
- Trauma – fat necrosis
- Abscess – lump almost always palpable.

Management of a breast lump

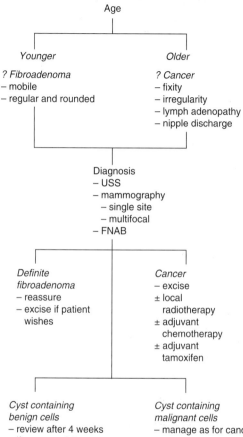

Age

Younger

? Fibroadenoma
– mobile
– regular and rounded

Older

? Cancer
– fixity
– irregularity
– lymph adenopathy
– nipple discharge

Diagnosis
– USS
– mammography
 – single site
 – multifocal
– FNAB

*Definite
fibroadenoma*
– reassure
– excise if patient
 wishes

Cancer
– excise
± local
 radiotherapy
± adjuvant
 chemotherapy
± adjuvant
 tamoxifen

*Cyst containing
benign cells*
– review after 4 weeks
– if reaccumulates,
 then reaspirate
– if continues to
 reaccumulate,
 then excise

*Cyst containing
malignant cells*
– manage as for cancer

Nipple discharge/change

Discharge This is not uncommon and is usually, but not always, benign. There are three common types:

* Milky   – pregnancy, lactation, prolactinoma
* Clear/greenish – mammillary fistula, duct ectasia
* Blood-stained – carcinoma, intraduct papilloma, Paget's disease of the nipple.

Sometimes discharge can be provoked by pressing on a 'trigger point' and this indicates the site of the underlying lesion.

Change A small number of diseases classically present with problems at the nipple:

* Paget's disease   – looks like eczema (underlying cancer)
* Nipple retraction – congenital (benign)
  benign (symmetrical, often both sides
  asymmetrical, older patient – ?cancer).

Changes in breast size

* Pregnancy
* Carcinoma
* Benign hypertrophy
* Giant fibroadenoma
* Phylloides tumour
* Sarcoma.

History

The history will be of the presenting complaint:

* What is wrong, when did you notice it, what has happened since?
* Then specific questions:
  – Lump (if not the presenting complaint)
  – Nipple discharge (if not the presenting complaint)
  – Pain (if not the presenting complaint)
  – Cyclical changes, changes with periods
  – Menstrual history (menarche, menopause, regularity)
  – Children, ?breast fed
  – Drugs (oral contraceptive, male gynaecomastia)
  – Family history of breast disease
  – Trauma, other symptoms…

Examination

What does the patient look like:

* old, young (fibroadenoma, cyst, cancer)
* well, ill, cachetic, pregnant.

Lump

* Arms up, behind head and down, look for asymmetry, etc.
* Size, site, side, shape, ulceration – where is it? (sitting up and lying down)

- Consistency, tenderness, lumpiness generally
- Fixity – superficial – pucker the skin for tethering, *p'eau d'orange*
  – deep – hands on hip, tense and relax, (NB The whole breast usually becomes less mobile with the pectoral muscles contracted so don't be deceived.)

Nipple

- Discharge – note the spot and send it for cytology
- Eczema – duct ectasia, Paget's disease of the nipple
- Retraction – symmetrical, bilateral...

Other specific examinations

- Other breast – examine this first
- Regional nodes – both axillae, supraclavicular and cervical

If possible malignancy:

- Abdomen – liver, ascites
- Chest – lung fields, skin nodules
- Spine – metastases to bone, tender spots
- Neuro – gait, etc. – cerebral metastases.

Investigation

Mammogram – recommended lowest age varies (usually 40 years), but getting younger
  – in every lump.

Lump

- FNAB and cytology (immediate is best):
  Fibroadenoma – feels hard (benign, abnormal cells)
  Cyst – green/brown fluid (lump disappears)
  Cancer – gritty feel (malignant abnormal cells)
  Ultrasound – sensitive for breast lumps, especially cysts.

Pain

- FNAB if well-localized area

Nipple

- Change – biopsy if possible Paget's disease
- Discharge – cytology.

Other specific tests

- Pregnancy – pregnancy test
- Probable malignancy – CXR, skeletal survey, bone scan, liver USS
  – FBC
  – U & E, LFT, calcium
  – Biopsy, hormone receptor expression.

Management

Details of management vary from centre to centre and are rapidly changing but the options are described here. Breast problems are best dealt with by a specialized team, including doctors, nurses and breast counsellors. This is particularly true of the management of breast cancer.

Lump

Fibroadenoma

- Prove by cytology – observe or excise
- Prove by excision biopsy.

Cyst

- Prove by aspiration – typical fluid and no lump – observe
  – bloody fluid and/or residual lump – mammography, cytology, excision biopsy.

Cancer

- Prove by cytology
- Account for patient preference, age and site/size/stage of disease
  Stage – T1S carcinoma in situ
  – T0 no evidence of primary tumour
  – T1 < 2 cm without fixation
  – T2 2–5 cm or < 2 cm with fixation
  – T3 5–10 cm
  – T4 extension to skin/chest wall or > 10 cm
  – N0 no nodes
  – N1 axillary – palpable but not clinically involved
  – clinically involved
  – N2 ipsilateral supraclavicular fossa
  – M0 no metastases
  – M1 distant metastases (includes contralateral axillary nodes)
  Treatment options include – lumpectomy + radiotherapy
  – mastectomy ± axillary surgery
  – endocrine therapy, tamoxifen, megace, oophorectomy
  – adrenalectomy, aminoglutethimide
  – radiotherapy
  – chemotherapy (single/multiple agents)
  Palliation – any of the above
  – analgesia for pain
  – paracentesis for effusions, ascites
  – corticosteroids
  – spironolactone
  – intracavity cytotoxics
  – specialized nursing care.

Pain

Breast pain is usually best managed by:

- Positive diagnosis – clinical, FNAB, mammogram
- Reassurance (provided benign)
- Simple analgesia (aspirin, paracetamol)
- Occasionally hormone therapy is needed
- Surgical treatment if very localized lump or abscess.

Nipple change/discharge

- Diagnosis – cytology, mammography
- Excision of specific lesion – intraduct papilloma, localized area of dysplasia
- Disconnection of duct if severe (Hadfield's procedure) – cannot breast feed afterwards.

ARTERIAL PROBLEMS

When clerking a patient with arterial disease always remember that the disease is unlikely to be localized to the presenting part, e.g. a patient with an aneurysm is also likely to have a degree of coronary artery and peripheral vascular disease. This may affect their pre- and postoperative care. You must also ask about risk factors for arterial disease such as smoking and diabetes mellitus because these are related to other disorders that may affect their intended operation.

Smoking-related disorders

- Chronic obstructive airways disease
- Bronchogenic carcinoma
- Peptic ulcer
- Other smoking-related neoplasia (oesophagus, stomach, bladder)
- Cardiac disease.

Diabetes-mellitus-related disorders

- Mixture of small and large vessel disease
- Renal disease (nephropathy)
- Retinopathy
- Autonomic neuropathy
- Peripheral neuropathy
- Infection
- Features of hyper- or hypoglycaemia (especially in starved or acutely ill patients).

Routine for assessing the arterial circulation

Inspection
Colour
   horizontal
   elevated
   dependent
Venous filling
Look at pressure areas and between digits.

Palpation
Skin temperature
Capillary refill time
Palpate the pulses.

Auscultation
Listen for bruits
Measure the blood pressure
Reactive hyperaemia time.

Management of arterial insufficiency

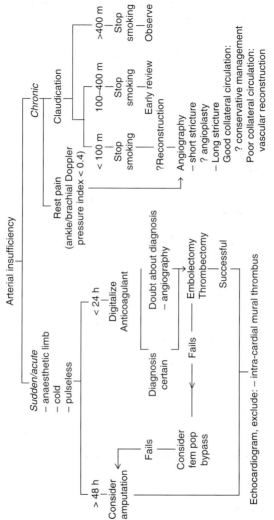

PERIPHERAL VASCULAR DISEASE (INTERMITTENT CLAUDICATION)

Symptoms

- Duration and progression of symptoms
- Claudication distance and recovery time
- Effect of weather, gradients, stairs
- Use of walking stick, heel raise
- Night pain, rest pain.

Signs

- Pulses
- Skin colour, temperature, presence of hair, ulcers
- Limb or digit loss
- Venous distension or guttering.

Effect of elevation followed by dependent position on limb skin colour (Buergher's test)

Buergher's test

Elevate the legs and look for venous guttering, blanching of the feet, especially the soles, and ask about calf pain (both can be hastened by asking the patient to plantar and dorsiflex the foot). The legs are then allowed to hang over the edge of the bed while you look for delayed venous filling followed by reactive hyperaemia.

ANEURYSMAL DISEASE

- Palpation of vessel diameter — expansile, not transmitted, pulsation
- Features of thrombosis — poor distal flow, especially if popliteal
- Features of embolus — pain, 'trash' foot
- Features of leakage — pain, bruising, swelling, hypotension.

THROMBOEMBOLIC DISEASE

Sudden onset of:

- Pain
- Pulselessness
- Perishing coldness
- Paraesthesia
- Pallor.

Usually associated with proximal source for embolism:

- Recent MI (mural thrombus)
- Atrial fibrillation
- Aneurysm.

Central disease:

- Angina
- Previous MI
- TIAs
- Stroke
- Mesenteric ischaemia.

Investigations

Bedside

> **Pressure index**
> Pressure index = Doppler pressure: ankle/brachial
> pressure
> >1 normal
> <1>0.7 mild claudication range
> <0.7>0.4 moderate claudication
> <0.4 limb at risk

- Feel all pulses and listen to all vessels
- Blood pressure in both arms and Doppler ankle pressure
- Vibration sense in diabetics (postganglionic C fibres – if lost then sympathectomy is no good).

Laboratory

- Ultrasound (vessel size and, with colour Doppler, flow)
- Blood studies:
  - FBC (polycythaemia, anaemia, viscosity clotting)
  - Blood sugar (diabetes), electrolytes (nephropathy)
- ECG (and stress test if angina is present)
- CXR (heart size and outline, COPD, bronchial carcinoma)
- X-ray diabetic feet:
  - Vessel calcification (tramline)
  - Gas in tissue (cellulitis not gas gangrene)
  - Osteomyelitis
- Arteriography (only if a decision to intervene has been made).

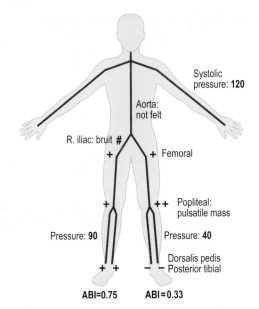

Fig 1.2 Investigations for arterial problems

THE VENOUS CASE

Varicose veins are usually due to sapheno-femoral incompetence. True short sapheno-politeal incompetence is much less common.

The aim is to identify the level of valvular incompetence by allowing high pressure deep venous blood to flow into low pressure saphenous vessels.

- Step 1: Mark all varicose veins (page 76)
- Step 2: Perform a Trendelenburg test:
  - Lie the patient supine, raise the leg to drain the veins and apply tourniquets at the mid-calf, just below the popliteal fossa, mid-thigh and just below the groin
  - Stand the patient up and remove the tourniquets serially from below, noting the level at which the veins suddenly fill (if you take too long to do this they will fill from below because of the normal circulation, so you have to be fairly quick to do the test accurately)

- Step 3: Identify perforators using Doppler ultrasound:
  - Place the Doppler probe over the perforator as demonstrated by the Trendelenberg test
  - Gently compress the calf repeatedly until the 'whoosh' of the venous blood is maximal
  - Mark this site
- Step 4: Venography. This is not a routine examination and is indicated when:
  - There is recurrence of complex varicose veins
  - After trauma, particularly in the postphlebitic syndrome (the superficial veins may be dilated because there are no patent deep veins)
  - Varicose veins following deep venous thrombosis
  - Short saphenous localization after failed surgery.

EXAMINATION OF AN ULCER

Look

- Site
- Size
- Shape
- Surface and depth
- Describe the edge (rolled, punched-out, peeling, clean)
- Describe the base (slough, exudate, visible structures).

Feel

- Texture of the edge
- Texture of the base
- Examine sensation
- Comment on regional lymph nodes and associated structures.

DYSPHAGIA

Dysphagia, or difficulty in swallowing, has dozens of potential causes but there are only four of practical importance to the surgeon. It may be due to mechanical or neuromuscular problems including *oesophageal spasm* and *achalasia*, but by far the most common causes of mechanical obstruction are *benign strictures* (secondary to reflux) and *carcinoma of the oesophagus*.

Potential causes of dysphagia

- Within the lumen:
  - Foreign body: typically a lump of meat. (NB. Sudden onset of dysphagia whilst eating nearly always occurs in an oesophagus which is already diseased, usually benign oesophageal stricture. People with a normal oesophagus can swallow swords, whole boiled eggs, pickled onions and other assorted large objects)
- Within the wall:
  - Inflammatory
    Peptic stricture: caused by reflux of stomach contents into the lower oesophagus
    Caustic stricture: caused by ingestion of irritant fluids, e.g. bleach, or tablets, e.g. slow-K, tetracycline
    Iatrogenic: caused by repeated sclerotherapy
  - Neoplastic
    Benign: lipoma, leiomyoma (rare)
    Malignant: adenocarcinoma, squamous carcinoma
  - Motility: scleroderma (stiffness of wall), spastic contractions ('corkscrew'), achalasia (failure of lower sphincter to relax), remote causes, e.g. motor neurone disease
- External compression:
  - Lymph nodes in mediastinum
  - Right atrium (heart failure)
  - Cervical osteophytes
  - Goitre.

History

- Where? (the site of dysphagia as perceived by the patient is usually above the anatomical site and rarely below it)
- How long?
- Progressive or intermittent?
- Solids or fluids?
- Weight loss?
- Other symptoms, e.g. heartburn, neurological disorder?

Examination

- Usually there are no abnormalities on examination
- Look out for signs of weight loss, supraclavicular lymphadenopathy and other diseases.

Management of dysphagia

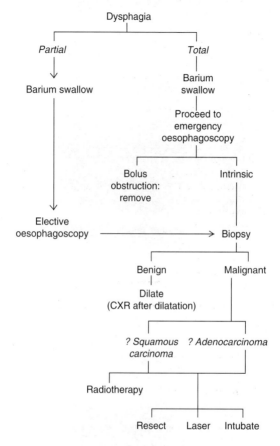

Investigations

- FBC (anaemia)
- U & E (dehydration/renal impairment)
- LFT (malignancy)
- CXR (aspiration, lymph nodes, fluid level)
- Barium swallow
  - A good first-line investigation
  - Ideal for the investigation of motility disorders
  - Sometimes desired by endoscopists prior to endoscopy
- Endoscopy
  - Benign-looking stricture: biopsy, dilatation (bougie, balloon)
  - Malignant-looking stricture: biopsy, dilatation (bougie), intubation, laser
  - Abnormal mucosa: biopsy (in suspected Barrett's, need four-quadrant biopsy), oesophagitis (grade it I).

Grades of oesophagitis

  I   = mucosal inflammation
  II = streaky ulceration
  III = circumferential ulceration
  IV = stenotic lesion, ulcer, Barrett's oesophagus

Following any oesophageal dilatation, always obtain a CXR to exclude oesophageal perforation.

Management

- *Intubation.* As well as endoscopic intubation (Atkinson tube), operative intubation of a malignant stricture of the oesophagus is possible through a gastrostomy performed at laparotomy.
- *Radiotherapy.* Squamous cell carcinoma is particularly sensitive to radiotherapy, which may be delivered either by external beam or from the lumen.
- *Surgery*
  Benign disease: confined to Heller's myotomy for achalasia and antireflux procedures of which there are at least 20 varieties
  Malignancy: oesophagectomy, which may be performed through abdominal, thoracic, cervical, laparoscopic or combined approaches.

THE JAUNDICED PATIENT

The clinical and biochemical picture in jaundice is often mixed. Obstructive jaundice may lead to secondary hepatocellular damage and the whole picture may be clouded by the features of the underlying cause (e.g. alcoholism or pancreatic cancer). Most patients admitted to surgical wards will have obstructive jaundice as their primary problem, since this is the only kind that is amenable to surgical treatment.

Specific features

Symptoms

- Jaundice (duration and progression of symptoms)
- Stool (pale) and urine colour (dark) (in obstructive jaundice)
- Pain, fever, rigors (pain + fever + jaundice = cholangitis; Charcot's triad)
- Malaise, weight loss (due to associated malignancy)
- Pruritis.

Signs

- Jaundice (sclera)
- Scratch marks
- Urine staining on underpants (due to bile pigments)
- Pale stool on PR.

Special investigations

- Urinalysis
- Electrolytes, LFTs (including conjugated and free bilirubin).

Secondary features

Symptoms

- Drug, alcohol and travel history
- Sexual history, i.v. drug abuse
- Biliary colic
- Weight loss, cachexia (malignancy, especially pancreatic)
- Previous malignant disease.

Signs

- Palpable gallbladder (Courvoisier's law)
- Epigastric mass (malignant nodes, pancreas)
- Ascites, encephalopathy, palmar erythema, flap, spider naevi (liver failure)
- Liver texture (knobbly – ?metastases; smooth, tender – ?hepatitis)
- Caput medusa, splenomegaly, anal varices (portal hypertension)

Management of a jaundiced patient

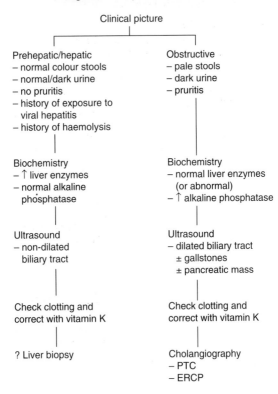

Clinical picture

Prehepatic/hepatic
– normal colour stools
– normal/dark urine
– no pruritis
– history of exposure to
  viral hepatitis
– history of haemolysis

Obstructive
– pale stools
– dark urine
– pruritis

Biochemistry
– ↑ liver enzymes
– normal alkaline
  phosphatase

Biochemistry
– normal liver enzymes
  (or abnormal)
– ↑ alkaline phosphatase

Ultrasound
– non-dilated
  biliary tract

Ultrasound
– dilated biliary tract
  ± gallstones
  ± pancreatic mass

Check clotting and
correct with vitamin K

Check clotting and
correct with vitamin K

? Liver biopsy

Cholangiography
– PTC
– ERCP

- Pyrexia, sweating, tachycardia (hepatitis, cholangitis)
- Hepatomegaly (cirrhosis, hepatitis).

Special investigations

- FBC (for anaemia or elevated white cell count)
- U & E (dehydration and renal impairment)
- Blood sugar
- Clotting screen, albumen (decreased hepatic function)
- Hepatitis viral antigen status
- Blood culture if pyrexial
- Ultrasound: duct dilatation, stones, pancreas, gallbladder, nodes
- Biliary imaging (ERCP or PTC), CT scan
- Angiography for hepatic or pancreatic resectional surgery
- Liver biopsy.
- Laparoscopy and laparoscopic ultrasound for staging of upper GI malignancy

---

Courvoisier's law

This is a misnomer (Courvoisier's hint might be better): Jaundice in the presence of a palpable gallbladder is unlikely to be due to stones (even if stones are present).

THE GROIN AND SCROTUM

For each inguinal hernia, examine the abdomen if this has not yet been done and look for anything that could have caused a rise in the intra-abdominal pressure, such as an enlarged prostate, ascites, pregnancy or chronic intestinal obstruction. Ask about chronic constipation and COPD.

Look

- Always examine the groin on both sides and the scrotum
- Look for normal scrotal development
- Look for a lump and a cough impulse and note site and direction
- Redness, sinuses, scars.

Feel

- Examine both testes (are both present?), epidiymi, and cords
- Tenderness (ask) and induration
- Palpate for cough impulse and note relationship to pubic tubercle (PT)
- Inguinal hernia above and medial to PT, femoral hernia below and lateral to PT
- Can you get above it?
- Can you feel the testis separate to it?

- Examine the lump for consistency, transilluminability
- Relationship to testis, i.e. above, below, or instead of (is it the testis?)
- Does it move separately or with the testis?
- For an undescended testis look for:
  - Associated hernia
  - Ectopic testis
  - Retractile testis
  - Bilateral arrested descent
  - Assess general development
  - Other congenital abnormalities.

CHANGE IN BOWEL HABIT

Change in bowel habit is a complaint that encompasses a large number of possible diagnoses. Patients may present because of a change in bowel habit or this may be a feature that is elicited by direct questioning after presentation with some other gastrointestinal symptom. What a patient considers to be normal will vary widely; the simple question, 'Are the bowels alright?', is not sufficient for a patient presenting with a gastrointestinal problem. Although the normal range for bowel habit is very wide, the patient's view of 'normal' may be very narrow and chronic use of laxatives (or, less commonly, constipating agents) is often because the patient wishes to achieve a particular bowel frequency that they regard as normal (twice round the pan, pointed at both ends and passed during the seven o'clock time signal on the radio!).

Change in frequency

The key here is *change* (Table 1.7). The normal variation in frequency of defaecation is huge and will range from several

Table 1.7
Change in bowel frequency

	Decrease	Increase
Change in diet:		
Decreased roughage	X	
Increased roughage		X
Peppers, chilli ...		X
Alcohol		X
Anorexia	X	
Malabsorption		X
Bowel inflammation		X
Obstruction	X	

Table 1.8
Change in stool consistency

	Harder	Looser
Bowel obstruction	X (usually)	X (sometimes)
Anorexia	X	
Bowel inflammation		X
Malabsorption		X
Roughage (increase)		X
Dehydration, hot weather	X	

times per day to once a week. If the patient has always had a regular bowel habit, whatever the frequency, and this *changes*, then this may indicate disease.

Change in consistency

As with frequency, *change* is the important factor (Table 1.8). The consistency of stools varies from individual to individual, from very loose to hard. Most people will attempt to rectify stool consistency if it is at the far end of the range because hard stools are hard to pass and very loose stools are thought to be abnormal.

Change in content or colour

Common changes in content are:

- Presence of mucus (IBD, malignancy)
- Presence of blood (malignancy, IBD, etc.).

Noticeable changes in colour are:

- Black stools (upper GI bleeding or oral iron therapy)
- White stools (obstructive jaundice or steatorrhoea).

2

Medical management of the surgical patient

MYOCARDIAL ISCHAEMIA

A past history of angina or MI is not an uncommon finding amongst patients admitted for elective surgical procedures. In a review of 1001 such procedures undertaken under general anaesthetic, Goldman et al (N Engl J Med 1977; 297: 845–50) found there were 19 postoperative cardiac deaths and 40 from non-cardiac causes. Cardiac complications after surgery occurred in 66 patients, of whom 18 had intra- or postoperative MI, 36 suffered cardiogenic pulmonary oedema and 12 had episodes of ventricular tachycardia. Multivariate analysis of preoperative findings suggested six important risk factors:

- Age > 70 years
- MI in the previous 6 months
- An S3 gallop rhythm or a raised JVP (S3 gallop rhythm is heard with a cadence best described by the phrase 'Kentucky, Kentucky, Kentucky')
- A rhythm other than sinus rhythm on the ECG
- > Five premature ventricular contractions/min documented at any time before surgery
- Significant aortic stenosis.

Using a cardiac risk index based mainly on these six criteria, patients with the fewest symptoms had a major complication rate of 1.6% after major surgery compared with a complication rate of 56% in those with four or more of the features listed above. Major complications were defined as MI, cardiogenic pulmonary oedema, ventricular tachycardia or cardiac death.

In view of the large differences in preoperative risk amongst patients with a previous cardiac history, it is important that they are carefully assessed before surgery. In addition to basic history, examination and investigation, it may frequently be necessary to obtain a cardiology opinion in order to optimize the patient's medical treatment and assess the risk of major surgery more formally.

ANGINA

History

1. Ascertain the frequency and severity of angina. The crucial differential is between stable and unstable angina. The

latter is defined as angina that is increasing in frequency and severity or occurs at rest.
2. Ascertain if the patient has had any associated symptoms, such as palpitations, shortness of breath or dependent oedema.
3. Make a careful list of the patient's medication, including how often they use their antianginals, e.g. GTN.

Examination

1. Examine the pulse, blood pressure, JVP and heart sounds. Listen for signs of pulmonary oedema.
2. In particular, listen for added heart sounds (3rd and 4th sounds). These are often difficult to detect, but the cadence of the heart rhythm with a 3rd sound is represented by 'Kentucky, Kentucky, Kentucky', and the cadence of the heart sounds when there is a 4th heart sound is represented by 'Tennessee, Tennessee, Tennessee'.
3. Check both sacrum and ankles for oedema.

Investigations

- FBC
- U & E
- ECG
- CXR.

Cardiology opinion

The aims of such a consultation are three-fold:

1. *To optimize the patient's medical treatment.* If the patient is not in heart failure, then myocardial work may be reduced by a combination of drugs:
   - Beta-blockers (slow the heart rate)
   - Nitrates (vasodilators)
   - Calcium channel antagonists, which may either act as vasodilators (as in the case of nifedipine) or to slow the heart rate (as in the case of verapamil).

   The aim of medication is to establish a resting heart rate of 60 bpm with a normal blood pressure of 130/70.
2. *To assess the preoperative risk.* This may be difficult and it is virtually impossible to give an exact percentage for the risk of cardiac complication or death. As mentioned above, risk scoring systems do exist, but a general rule is that patients who can carry two plastic carrier bags loaded with shopping up a single flight of stairs without stopping, or without chest pain, will tolerate most surgery well.
3. *To institute further investigation.* If the patient is felt to be at high risk of myocardial complications, further investigation by echocardiogram, exercise tolerance test, or thallium or technetium-gated cardiac scanning may better assess myocardial perfusion and performance.

MYOCARDIAL INFARCTION

Many patients who come to hospital for elective surgery will have had an MI in the past. Obviously, a patient who suffered a small MI 10 years previously, is not on regular medication, and has no residual symptoms can be regarded as low risk for major surgery. In the presence of other symptoms suggesting cardiac failure or an MI within the previous 6 months, the risk of postoperative complications increases. Preoperative assessment is aimed at picking up such features with a view to optimizing medication and, if necessary, delaying surgery to avoid undue risk.

History

1. Clarify the number and time of previous MI and, if possible, obtain hospital notes describing those admissions.
2. Check for current symptoms of angina, palpitations, shortness of breath or oedema.
3. Note regular medication.

Examination

As for a patient with angina (see page 48).

Investigations (see also page 49)

As for a patient with angina (see page 48).

Cardiology opinion

The aims of a cardiology opinion are two-fold:

1. *To adjust medication to optimize myocardial function.* This may include increasing treatment for heart failure (diuretics, ACE inhibitors).
2. *Routine assessment,* especially after a recent infarct, which may include exercise tolerance test, echocardiogram, thallium scan and assessment of ventricular function using a technetium-gated radioisotope scan.

Broad guidelines about surgery after MI

- Purely elective surgery should be delayed at least 6 months.
- Semi-urgent surgery, e.g. for malignancy, should be delayed for at least 6 weeks.
- Emergency surgery, e.g. for life-threatening GI haemorrhage, may need to be undertaken immediately in any case.
- In all cases, intensive anaesthetic monitoring of tissue oxygenation, blood gases, electrolytes, circulating volume and haematocrit are essential to minimize postoperative cardiac complications.

CARDIAC ARREST

Usually a cardiac arrest will be managed by the 'arrest team' made up of an SHO in medicine and a second SHO in anaesthesia. Occasionally, however, you will be the first person at a cardiac arrest and it is therefore important to proceed in an appropriate fashion until the 'team' arrives.

1. Assess responsiveness and breathing, and check that the carotid pulse is absent: this confirms the diagnosis.
2. *Call the 'crash team'*, check the time and ask for the resuscitation and defibrillator trolley.
3. Start CPR, give a precordial thump: this may terminate ventricular arrhythmias.
4. Place patient on the floor or a hard board. Open *airway:* ensure head tilt and chin lift; check *breathing*; close nose and give two breaths, alternated with 15 chest compressions if carotid pulse absent (at a rate of about 80 compressions/min).
5. Defibrillate as soon as possible with DC 200 J.
6. When help arrives, *delegate*:
   – Ask someone to give 100% oxygen with an ambu-bag
   – Ask someone to put up a central line or i.v. line
   – ask the anaesthetist or insert yourself an endotracheal tube
   – Place ECG leads.

If the patient is in VF or pulseless VT

1. Give a precordial thump and first DC shock 200 J if not yet given
   – Recharge, check pulse and ECG monitor for 5 s.
2. Give second DC shock 200 J
   – Recharge, check pulse and ECG monitor for 5 s.
3. Give third DC shock 360 J.
4. Give i.v. access and intubate if not already done, and give 1 mg adrenaline i.v.
5. 10 CPR sequences of 5:1 compression/ventilation.
6. DC shock 360 J.
7. DC shock 360 J.
8. DC shock 360 J.
9. Repeat steps (4) to (8) for as long as defibrillation is indicated.
10. After three cycles, consider alkalizing and antiarrhythmic agents.

If the patient is in asystole

1. Precordial thump.
2. Exclude VF, give i.v. access and intubate if not already done, and give 1 mg adrenaline i.v.
3. 10 CPR sequences of 5:1 compression/ventilation.

4. Atropine 3 mg i.v. once only.
5. Repeat steps (2) and (3) if electrical activity not evident.
6. If no response after three cycles, consider high-dose adrenaline 5 mg i.v.

If the patient is in pulseless electrical activity (PEA, formerly termed electromechanical dissociation)

1. Think of and, if indicated, give specific treatment for:
   - Electrolyte imbalance
   - Drug overdose/intoxication
   - Hypothermia
   - Hypovolaemia
   - Tension pneumothorax
   - Cardiac tamponade
   - Pulmonary embolism.
2. Give i.v. access and intubate if not already done, and give 1 mg adrenaline i.v.
3. 10 CPR sequences of 5:1 compression/ventilation.
4. Repeat steps (2) and (3) if no pulse.

Remember

- The patient should be pink and perfused during resuscitation. If not, ventilation may be inadequate (check the oxygen has not run out and the endotracheal tube is correctly placed) or the patient's collapse may be due to pulmonary causes, e.g. a pulmonary embolus or pneumothorax.
- Check the patient's pupils. If dilating, or fixed and dilated, brain damage has probably occurred.

HYPERTENSION

Raised blood pressure, both treated and untreated, is a common finding in patients admitted for elective surgery. In 676 consecutive operations in patients over 40, Goldman et al (Anaesthesiology 1979;50:285–92) studied pre, intra- and postoperative blood pressure.

A multivariate analysis of these groups of patients revealed that increased blood pressure in itself was not a predisposing factor to myocardial ischaemia or infarction, renal failure or blood pressure lability during or after surgery. It was therefore concluded that patients with mild to moderate hypertension (diastolic pressure < 110 mmHg), who also had no evidence of serious end-organ damage, were generally fit for a major operation under general anaesthetic. Furthermore, antihypertensive medication should be continued up to the day of surgery.

From this study it is clear that preoperative assessment should highlight patients who are either severely hypertensive (diastolic pressure > 110 mmHg), or have end-organ damage, including hypertensive retinopathy or nephropathy.

History

The majority of patients with hypertension are asymptomatic and routine history is often unhelpful. There may, however, be symptoms related to end-organ damage, such as shortness of breath, angina or peripheral oedema.

Examination

In addition to routine examination, be careful to check the patient's blood pressure yourself. Make sure the patient is sitting and at rest. If the blood pressure is marginally raised:

1. Wait half an hour and recheck it.
2. Listen for the presence of a 4th heart sound (cadence 'Tennessee, Tennessee, Tennessee').
3. Check carefully the position of the cardiac apex and the nature of the beat, which may be 'thrusting' in cases of left ventricular hypertrophy.
4. Examine the eyes looking for hypertensive retinopathy.
5. Examine all peripheral pulses and, in particular, listen for signs of a carotid bruit.
6. Dip a routine urine sample to test for protein.

Investigations

- FBC
- U & E
- ECG
- CXR.

Cardiology opinion

If you or the anaesthetist are concerned about the patient's hypertension, a cardiology opinion may be sought. The purposes of this are two-fold:

1. *To check for complications of hypertension.*
2. *To optimize the patient's medication in preparation for surgery.*
   Four basic types of medication are used in the treatment of hypertension:
   – Beta-blockers
   – Diuretics (mainly thiazide with or without the addition of a potassium-sparing diuretic, such as amiloride)
   – Calcium antagonists
   – ACE inhibitors.

As already stated, patients with mild to moderate hypertension with no evidence of end-organ damage are not at increased risk from major surgery. However, patients with more severe hypertension or with signs of end-organ damage may require alteration of their medication in order to prepare them for major surgery.

RESPIRATORY DISEASE

You will often be faced with patients who have longstanding respiratory disease and need either urgent or elective surgery. If the surgery is for a life-threatening emergency, then pre-existing respiratory disease is unlikely to affect the decision to operate. However, in the case of elective surgery, preoperative medical treatment and intraoperative care can greatly reduce the postoperative morbidity suffered by patients with a pre-existing respiratory disorder.

CHRONIC OBSTRUCTIVE PULMONARY DISEASE

This is the most commonly encountered chronic respiratory disease. In patients with chronic obstructive pulmonary disease, increased sputum production will predispose to postoperative atelectasis and pneumonia. Patients with severe disease are liable to develop respiratory failure due to the increased work of breathing, the decrease in respiratory drive after surgery and defective pulmonary gas exchange.

ASTHMA

Patients with asthma who are in remission present very few problems to the anaesthetist. Most general anaesthetic agents have a mild bronchodilator effect; this is supplemented by the catecholamine and corticosteroid output at the time of surgery which may also improve bronchodilatation. Patients on long-term corticosteroids for asthma should receive their usual medication on the morning of surgery and have their operation covered by hydrocortisone 100 mg q.d.s. i.v. In addition, it may be wise to add a salbutamol nebulizer to the premedication.

INTERSTITIAL LUNG DISEASE

Patients with interstitial lung disease have diffuse pulmonary fibrosis from various causes, and this leads to impaired gas exchange. In general, such patients do not experience problems during general anaesthesia and any tendency to hypoxia can be compensated for by increasing the oxygen concentration in the inspired gas during general anaesthesia.

CHEST WALL AND MUSCLE DISEASE

Patients who are unable to inspire deeply because of restrictive chest wall disease, such as in ankylosing spondylitis or skeletal muscle paralysis, e.g. poliomyelitis, are at risk of increased pulmonary problems after general anaesthesia. Postoperatively they may have problems coughing adequately and may therefore find it difficult to clear the large airways. The sedative effects of general anaesthetic and postoperative analgesia may tip such patients over into respiratory failure and this may make it extremely difficult to wean them from the ventilator.

History/examination

1. Recognize patients with impaired pulmonary function.
2. Ask specifically about symptoms of breathlessness, cough, sputum production and smoking.
3. In particular, assess severity of dyspnoea and exercise tolerance and ask specifically about the nature of sputum (purulent or clear).

Investigations

- CXR – this will exclude unexpected underlying pulmonary disease, e.g. pneumonia, an unsuspected bronchial carcinoma or a pneumothorax in an asthmatic patient.
- Microscopy and culture of sputum specimen – this will allow an organism to be isolated in the presence of acute infection and antibiotic sensitivities to be determined.
- Simple pulmonary function tests – using a vitalograph, the fixed vital capacity and FEV_1 can be measured. If the FEV_1 is < 1 litre or 50% of the predicted value for that patient, then blood gases should also be estimated.
- ABGs.
- FBC – to reveal polycythaemia due to chronic hypoxia or a raised white cell count secondary to respiratory infection.
- U & E – particularly important in patients who may have been receiving long-term diuretics.

Fitness for surgery

In spite of a large amount of work studying pulmonary function tests in patients before major surgery, it is difficult to give hard and fast rules about who is fit for surgery and who is not. In general, however:

- Patients with a low PaO_2 or dyspnoea at rest will often require postoperative ventilation.
- Patients with an FEV_1 of <1 litre will often require postoperative ventilation.
- Patients with a PaO_2 of <6 kPa will often require ventilation postoperatively even if they are not short of breath at rest

Effects of a general anaesthetic on respiratory function

Premedication

A patient's premed often contains an anticholinergic drug such as atropine, and an opioid with or without the addition of a sedative, which is often from the benzodiazepine group of drugs. Anticholinergic drugs make bronchial secretions thicker but also have a mild bronchodilator effect and, on balance, have very little impact on respiratory function. Both opiates and benzodiazepines, however, have the side-effect of respiratory depression and in patients who are already hypoxic they may exacerbate respiratory disease.

General anaesthesia

General anaesthesia itself reduces the respiratory drive for a given end-tidal CO_2 and, as such, leads to impaired respiratory function. General anaesthetics also depress the hypoxic ventilatory response. Thus in a postoperative patient, the drive to breathe in response to a raised PCO_2 or lowered PO_2 will be depressed. In addition, intubation and the administration of a general anaesthetic impair mucociliary clearance, which may lead to increased sputum retention. A third, and as important effect of general anaesthesia, is its impact on the functional residual capacity, which leads to collapse (atelectasis) at the bases of both lungs. This, together with impaired coughing, impaired mucociliary clearance and reduced respiratory drive, may lead to postoperative chest infections.

Postoperative complications

- *Sputum retention* secondary to impaired coughing and mucociliary clearance.
- *Hypoxaemia* secondary to sedative effects of a general anaesthetic.
- *Atelectasis* and *bronchopneumonia* as a result of the above. Bronchopneumonia is particularly common when there is pre-existing chronic respiratory infection, which is exacerbated by basal collapse in the lungs.
- *Respiratory failure.* In some patients with severe COPD, the combined deleterious effects of a general anaesthetic will lead to respiratory failure. In such cases, the patient may need artificial ventilation for anything between a few hours and few days postoperatively, but it is usually possible to wean them from the ventilator as long as there are no other major postoperative pulmonary complications

ENDOCRINE CONDITIONS

DIABETES

There are over half a million diabetics in Great Britain, so it is not uncommon for you to be presented with a diabetic requiring elective or emergency surgery. Complications of diabetes predispose this group to increased vascular, ophthalmic and renal surgery.

Remember

When thinking about diabetic patients:

- Diabetic patients are more prone to vascular, renal and ophthalmic disease.
- The stress of surgery causes the release of hormones antagonistic to the actions of insulin, e.g. adrenaline, ACTH/cortisol, glucagon and growth hormone. This can result in a deterioration of diabetic control.
- The stress of surgery may therefore cause latent diabetes to be unmasked and stable diabetes to become unstable.
- The metabolic consequences of stress and insulin antagonism include an increase in gluconeogenesis, contributing to hyperglycaemia, increased lipolysis, a risk of ketosis and a predisposition to lactic acidosis.
- Hyperglycaemia also contributes to hyperviscosity and hyperosmolality, leading to increased osmotic diuresis and dehydration.
- Hyperglycaemia and dehydration increase the risk of venous thrombosis.
- Hyperglycaemia impairs phagocyte function and increases the risk of infection and delayed wound healing.

TREATMENT OF THE PATIENT WITH DIABETES (IDDM AND NIDDM)

Before admission

1. Treat obesity.
2. Discuss the consequences of smoking for a diabetic surgical patient.
3. Assess if glycaemia controlled:
   - Random blood glucose <12 mmol/l
   - Fasting blood glucose <8 mmol/l
   - HbA_1 <10%
   - No hypoglycaemia.

4. Substitute:
   – Long-acting sulphonylureas (chlorpropamide and glibenclamide) by gliclazide or tolbutamide
   – Long-acting insulins (Human Ultratard) by intermediate-acting formulations.
5. Ensure adequate treatment of ischaemic heart disease.
6. Ensure adequate treatment of hypertension.
7. Look for autonomic neuropathy (dysrhythmias, orthostatic hypotension, delayed gastric emptying, impotence, sweating): alert anaesthetist.
8. Look for peripheral neuropathy: alert nurses (bedsores on heels).

During admission

1. Fast the patient as usual before surgery.
2. Ensure patient is first on operation list.
3. Control diabetes in accordance with Table 2.1.
4. Monitor BG every 2 hours (BM Stix).
5. Check potassium at 4 h, 8 h and, if stable, every 24 h after that.
6. Change insulin by 4 units per bag if BG <6 mmol/l or >12 mmol/l.
7. When the patient is able to eat solid food: give subcutaneous insulin or oral therapy, feed the patient and discontinue GKI.

Table 2.1
Control of diabetes

	Minor surgery	Major surgery
Well-controlled NIDDM (FBG <8 mmol/l)	1. Omit oral antidiabetic drugs 2. Avoid glucose-containing fluids 3. Monitor blood glucose (BG) 4. Restart oral therapy when patient ready to eat	GKI
Poorly controlled NIDDM	GKI	GKI
IDDM	GKI	GKI

GKI = 10% dextrose 500 ml, 16 units Actrapid and 10 mmol KCl at a rate of 100 ml/h.

8. If the patient is unable to eat within 48 h, make sure that a saline infusion is also given to prevent hyponatraemia.
9. If BG >17 mmol/l, change to a continuous insulin infusion (500 ml of normal saline, 30 units Actrapid, 10 mmol KCl) at a rate of 6 units/h until BG <12 mmol/l.
10. If BG <4 mmol/l, run in 100 ml 10% dextrose, recheck BG and continue GKI.

> **Remember**
>
> Poor glycaemic control may lead to delayed wound healing and increased postoperative infection. In addition, diabetic patients who are hypertensive or have ischaemic heart disease, have increased postoperative cardiovascular complications. Patients with an autonomic neuropathy are an anaesthetic hazard and are particularly at risk of pressure sores.

Special cases (discuss with anaesthetist)

1. Less insulin required (12 units/bag)
   – If total daily subcutaneous dose <30 units
   – Previous pancreatectomy patient.
2. More insulin required (20 units/bag)
   – Total daily subcutaneous dose >80 units
   – Marked obesity
   – Steroid dependent
   – Acromegaly.
3. Extremely high insulin requirements
   – Cardiopulmonary bypass surgery.
4. Small volume of fluid is required (use 20% dextrose)
   – In chronic renal failure patients.

Postoperative emergencies

High blood sugar

If a raised BG is an isolated result, repeat the BM Stix and if it is still raised:

1. Adjust the insulin dose in the GKI.
2. Check the urine for ketones.
3. Take a history, examine the patient and investigate appropriately to look for infection in case this is the cause of their increased insulin requirement.

Low blood sugar

In a patient where the BM Stix has shown hypoglycaemia:

1. Check for symptoms of hypoglycaemia (sweating, tachycardia, confusion).
2. If the patient is hypoglycaemic, increase their glucose immediately but do not stop the insulin infusion.

3. If they have no symptoms of hypoglycaemia then recheck the BM Stix.

Patient fitting

A patient who has an epileptic-like seizure in the postoperative period is invariably hypoglycaemic. When you are called to see them:

1. Ensure that the patient's airway is clear and that there is intravenous access.
2. Check the BM Stix from the intravenous access site and send a parallel sample to the biochemistry laboratory for more accurate glucose estimation (see page 268)
3. Temporarily stop the insulin infusion if it is running and administer 50 ml of 50% glucose rapidly i.v.
4. If the fit is not controlled by the administration of i.v. glucose within 2 min, give 5–10 mg of diazepam i.v.
5. Consider the infusion of 10% glucose without insulin if the patient does not appear to improve or their BG returns to the normal range.

Patient drowsy, irritable or aggressive

Again, this is probably due to hypoglycaemia and should be managed as for a patient fitting by checking the BM Stix, increasing the glucose and reviewing the insulin administration.

Key points in the management of a diabetic patient during surgery

- Adequate preoperative blood glucose control.
- Adequate glucose monitoring by BM Stix during hospital admission.
- Preoperative blood pressure evaluation and ECG to spot dangerous cardiovascular disease.
- Place the patient first on the list and inform the anaesthetist and medical team in advance that there is a diabetic patient who requires surgery.

THYROTOXICOSIS

This poses a serious anaesthetic risk because of the increased incidence of MI, cardiac arrhythmia and embolic phenomena in such patients.

Remember

Thyrotoxicosis can present in many ways and can mimic other conditions with weight loss, anorexia, nausea, diarrhoea and embolic disease as presenting features.

History

Ask specifically about palpitations, sweating, recent mood changes, preference for hot or cold weather, weight loss, increased appetite, change in bowel habit or any other recent illness.

Examination

1. Check the pulse and blood pressure.
2. Examine the eyes for signs of lid lag.
3. Examine the neck for signs of thyroid nodule or thyroid bruit.

Investigations

- Elevated T3 and T4, low TSH
- Autoantibodies
- Thyroid radioisotope scan.

Management

A thyrotoxic patient should *never* go to theatre unrecognized. If surgery is unavoidable, rapid institution of adequate beta-blockade is mandatory, if not contraindicated for some other reason. Even 24 h of high-dose beta-blockade using propranolol up to 40 mg q.d.s. will help greatly. Not only does beta-blockade reduce the tachycardia and risk of arrhythmia in thyrotoxicosis, but it also inhibits the conversion peripherally of T4 into T3.

Having recognized the patient is thyrotoxic, a medical referral is indicated for two reasons:

1. *To investigate the patient.* A major differential diagnosis of patients with thyrotoxicosis is a toxic multinodule goitre or autoimmune thyroid disease, e.g. Grave's disease. Investigation proceeds by taking blood for autoantibodies and arranging a thyroid technetium–99m scan.
2. *To treat the patient*:
   - *Medical treatment*: after 2–3 weeks treatment with high-dose carbimazole and beta-blockers add thyroxin (T4). Medical treatment is usually continued for 1 year and then withdrawn to see if the patient's thyrotoxicosis relapses.
   - *Surgical treatment*: usually in the form of sub-total thyroidectomy. The aim of such a procedure is to reduce the functioning mass of the thyroid and thereby reverse the hyperthyroidism
   - *Radioiodine*: generally used in patients over 60 years of age and in whom medical treatment has failed and surgery is contraindicated.

HYPOADRENALISM

This may be either primary or secondary to pituitary insufficiency. Such patients have invariably already been diagnosed and are on life-long replacement therapy with glucocorticoids and mineralocorticoids. The management of such a patient on a surgical ward, therefore, predominantly involves the control of their steroid therapy during their surgical admission.

Causes of primary hypoadrenalism include autoimmune disease, secondary carcinoma and tuberculosis; however, it is important to remember that potent antiendocrine drugs, such as aminoglutethimide, have the same effect as a surgical adrenalectomy. In addition, some drugs, such as ketoconazole which is given for fungal infections, may exacerbate the hypoadrenalism caused by aminoglutethimide. As a general rule, anyone on long-term steroids, or who has come off them in the last 6 months, should be assumed to be potentially steroid dependent, or have an impaired stress response. All such patients should be managed in the following fashion.

Minor operative procedures, e.g. cystoscopy

1. Continue normal oral steroids up until the morning of surgery.
2. Give hydrocortisone 100 mg i.v. or i.m. 1 h preoperatively.

Intermediate procedures, e.g. hernia repair

1. Continue normal oral steroids up until the morning of surgery.
2. Commence hydrocortisone 100 mg i.v. 1 h before surgery and continue at 6-hourly intervals for 24 h.

Major surgery

1. Continue normal oral steroids up until the morning of surgery.
2. Commence hydrocortisone 100 mg i.v. 1 h before surgery and continue at 6-hourly intervals for 72 h.
3. After 72 h of hydrocortisone reintroduce the patient's normal oral steroid therapy.
4. Add to this, hydrocortisone 20 mg orally t.d.s. and gradually reduce this dose over the next 2–3 weeks depending on the condition of the patient.

Postoperative emergencies

Any subsequent medical emergency after surgery, such as an MI, will need a doubling of the usual dose of hydrocortisone orally or parenterally.

Signs of inadequate steroid replacement

- Tachycardia
- Hypotension
- Nausea
- Pyrexia.

ACUTE RENAL INSUFFICIENCY

Acute renal insufficiency may be caused by a rapid decrease in glomerular filtration rate, usually secondary to reduced renal perfusion (sepsis, haemorrhage), or nephrotoxic injury (drugs, sepsis, bilirubin – hepatorenal syndrome). This rapid decrease in glomerular filtration rate leads to:

- A rise in serum urea and creatinine
- Reduced or absent urine output
- Volume expansion with oedema, hypotension and ultimately congestive cardiac failure
- Hyperkalaemia, dilutional hyponatraemia and acidosis.

Both prerenal and postrenal causes of acute renal failure are potentially reversible and it is therefore important to ensure:

- Adequate renal perfusion
- Exclusion of ureteric, urethral or catheter obstruction.

Management of acute renal failure in the postoperative patient is discussed on page 91.

CHRONIC RENAL INSUFFICIENCY

Some degree of chronic renal impairment is common amongst elderly patients presenting for routine surgery. Chronic renal insufficiency is defined as a raised urea or creatinine for >3 months and may be associated with bilaterally shrunken kidneys, hypertension, oedema, polyuria or oliguria. In patients with chronic renal insufficiency the most important consideration is to avoid fluid overload and, if possible, avert any rapid fluctuations in blood pressure which might exacerbate renal failure. In all cases, when a patient is discovered to have a raised urea or creatinine, careful history, examination and simple investigation should be undertaken to establish whether their chronic renal failure is stable or unstable.

History

1. Check for symptoms of polyuria or oliguria.
2. Establish in the past medical history whether the patient is diabetic or has had previous glomerular nephritis.
3. Check whether the patient has had previous outflow obstruction or a previous transurethral prostatectomy.

Examination

1. Check blood pressure.
2. Examine the abdomen for any abnormal renal swelling.

3. Check for a palpable or percussable bladder.
4. Check for prostatic hypertrophy or pelvic masses by rectal examination.

Investigations

- Perform a simple dipstick test on the urine to check for protein.
- U & E – in addition to looking for raised urea and creatinine, check for raised K^+ or low Na^+.
- ABGs may be required if you suspect the patient is acidotic.

Management

Stable chronic renal insufficiency

- In a patient where there is evidence of longstanding mild renal impairment (creatinine <200 mmol/l), there is no contraindication to general surgery.
- Nephrotoxic drugs such as gentamicin are contraindicated in such patients and it is generally safer to avoid them completely rather than administer a lower dose.
- All patients with chronic renal impairment require a CVP line placed preoperatively (see page 179) and retained for 24–48 h postoperatively to ensure they are not fluid overloaded.

Progressive chronic renal failure

It is often difficult to know beyond reasonable doubt that a patient has chronic renal insufficiency, particularly if no U & E measurements have been performed during the previous 12 months. In general, a patient does not require further investigation and should be managed in the same fashion as a patient known to have stable chronic renal insufficiency if:

- no symptoms of chronic renal failure
- creatinine <200 mmol/l
- normal serum Na^+ and K^+
- not acidotic
- no proteinuria
- over 70 years of age.

Conversely, in a patient who has symptoms of renal failure, or in whom the creatinine is raised or the U & E deranged, it may be wise to refer them to a nephrologist for further renal investigations.

Nephrology referral   The aim is to facilitate further study of the kidneys by four means:

1. Abdominal ultrasound – to look at the physical characteristics of the kidneys.
2. Intravenous urogram – to look at both the function of the kidney and the urinary outflow tract.

3. Isotope renogram – to assess blood flow to the kidneys.
4. Creatinine clearance – to measure renal function.

A nephrology referral may highlight reversible pathology, such as renovascular disease, which may merit treatment by interventional radiology or surgery prior to another surgical procedure. Alternatively, progressive renal disease, such as glomerulonephritis, may benefit from medical intervention.

HEPATIC INSUFFICIENCY

The most frequent problem leading to surgical admission for patients with hepatic insufficiency is haemorrhage from oesophageal varices. The most common cause of hepatic insufficiency is cirrhosis secondary to chronic alcohol abuse, although a variety of other conditions may also cause cirrhosis (viral hepatitis, hepatotoxic drugs and rarer conditions such as Wilson's disease and haemochromatosis).

History/examination
Hepatic insufficiency may present in a number of ways and whilst taking a history and examining the patient it is important to look out for symptoms and signs of the nine methods of presentations:

- Neuropsychiatric – stupor, delirium, coma
- Cerebral oedema – irritability, decerebrate rigidity
- Progressive jaundice
- Coagulopathy and bleeding
- Hypoglycaemia
- Acute renal failure
- Pancreatitis
- Sepsis
- Cardiopulmonary overload.

Investigations

- FBC – anaemia or sepsis
- U & E – renal failure, raised sodium
- Glucose – hypoglycaemia
- Amylase – pancreatitis
- Clotting – coagulopathy and haemorrhage
- Group blood and save for cross-match – in case of haemorrhage.

Management

- Maintain the airway. Many patients have a reduced level of consciousness which may fluctuate and it is important to ensure that they have patent airways at all times.

- Correct any hypoglycaemia without volume overload – use 10 or 20% dextrose.
- Minimize sodium input – this means avoiding all saline infusions.

> **Remember**
>
> Many antibiotics are made up of sodium salts. A patient once recorded a sodium of 186 mmol/l despite receiving no intravenous saline. The sole cause of this raised sodium was the administration of the penicillin sodium salt for an infection associated with hepatic failure.

- Prevent GI haemorrhage. Proton pump inhibitors or an H_2 receptor antagonist may be used in addition to mucosal protectants such as sucralfate 1 g q.d.s.
- Correct clotting disorders. This may be undertaken using a combination of parenteral vitamin K and fresh frozen plasma.
- Avoid anticoagulant drugs, e.g. aspirin.
- Avoid hepatotoxic drugs, e.g. paracetamol.
- Avoid drugs that require hepatic metabolism as part of their elimination, e.g. opiates.

> **Remember**
>
> Naloxone, the opiate antagonist, only acts for between 30 and 45 min and in patients with severely impaired hepatic function, it may be necessary to set up a continuous infusion.

- Minimize the bacterial content of the bowel. This is accomplished using a laxative, such as lactulose 20 ml b.d. or magnesium sulphate, and a topically active antibiotic such as neomycin.
- If the patient is in incipient renal failure, consider the use of mannitol 300 ml over 30 min.
- Ascites, which is common in hepatic failure, may be managed using a combination of spironolactone 100 mg b.d. and frusemide 20–80 mg b.d. Draining hepatic ascites is dangerous and will cause circulatory collapse. A small diagnostic tap is perfectly safe, but removing 2–3 litres of proteinaceous fluid will simply be followed by the formation of further protein-rich ascites, which will further deplete the circulating volume of the patient.

3

The operating list

67

Your job is to admit patients to the hospital and, in the majority of surgical cases, prepare them for an operation. However, there are cases under the care of a surgeon who are admitted only for investigation or non-operative treatment. In addition there are surgical patients whose treatment can now be undertaken endoscopically or by the interventional radiologist.

Operations will be performed either electively on a routine designated list or as an emergency, either out of hours or on an open emergency list. Essentially their preoperative work-up is very similar, except that in the emergency situation there may also be the need for some form of resuscitation (see pages 2, 88).

ELECTIVE SURGERY

The day of admission
Clerk the patients, with specific regard to:

- Confirming the diagnosis
- Any new problems since they were last seen in the clinic
- Fitness for anaesthesia: pulmonary and cardiovascular status (always check the blood pressure and urine) (see pages 10, 33, 48, 52, 63)
- Current medical problems and drug therapy
- Allergies, particularly antibiotics, iodine and elastoplast
- Problems with previous surgery and anaesthesia, particularly DVT
- Smoking
- Explain the procedure or operation to the patient, and obtain written consent from the patient, parent or guardian (see page 108).

Investigations may be *general* (relating to anaesthesia) and *specific* (relating to the patient's disease or proposed operation).

General investigations

- FBC (see page 260)
  - All patients undergoing general anaesthesia
- Sickle (see page 260)
  - All non-Caucasian patients undergoing general anaesthesia
- Thalassaemia
  - All patients of Mediterranean origin who are anaemic
- Clotting screen
  - All patients undergoing major surgery
  - All jaundiced patients
  - Patients on long-term anticoagulation or with a history of thromboembolic disease
- Biochemistry (U & E, SMAC) (see page 268)
  - All patients over 40 years of age

- All patients undergoing major surgery
- All patients with cardiac, pulmonary or renal disease (including obstructive uropathy due to prostatism)
- All jaundiced patients
- All patients who are clinically dehydrated
- All patients on diuretic therapy
- All diabetics
- All patients with a pituitary–adrenal axis syndrome

- Blood sugar
  - All diabetics
- Liver function
  - Patients with current or recent jaundice
  - All patients undergoing hepatobiliary surgery
- CXR
  - Patients with a history of respiratory disease (including recent chest infection/productive cough)
  - All patients listed for major surgery, especially resection of malignancy and thoracic surgery
  - All smokers undergoing a general anaesthetic
- ECG
  - All patients over the age of 50 years
  - All patients suspected of cardiac disease.

Specific investigations

These are listed in Table 3.1. In general:

- Blood group and save or cross-match – all major surgery should be blood grouped. In addition, specific large-scale operations should have blood cross-matched.
- Respiratory function tests and ABGs – all patients who will have their chest opened as part of their surgery. In addition, any patient coming to surgery with either a respiratory or metabolic acid–base problem (e.g. renal failure, pyloric stenosis) (see page 63).
- Special requests for intraoperative radiology and/or ultrasound (X-ray). If intraoperative imaging is required, particularly in orthopaedic, vascular access and biliary procedures, this will have to be arranged and organized through the radiology department the day before surgery
- Frozen-section histological examination. As a rule, notify the histology department of any cancer surgery that is scheduled for the next day's operating list

Special arrangements

Most operations require no further preparation. However, a number of operations require specific arrangements or procedures before they can be performed:

- Arranging an intensive therapy (ITU) bed. All cardiothoracic, major vascular and large GI resectional operations should be undertaken with an ITU bed available. This should be arranged with the Consultant in charge of ITU as far in advance as is feasible.

Table 3.1
Operation planner for common major operations

Operation	FBC	SMAC	CXR	ECG	Clotting	G&S/XM
Breast surgery						
Simple mastectomy	X	X	X	X	X	X
Radical mastectomy	X	X	X	X	X	X
Breast reconstruction	X	X	X	X	X	2
Cardiothoracic surgery						
Oesophageal dilatation	X	X	X	X	X	X
Oesophagectomy (all types)	X	X	X	X	X	4
Oesophageal transection (varices)	X	X	X	X	X	6
Oesophageal atresia surgery	X	X	X		X	2
Thoracotomy	X	X	X	X	X	2
Pulmonary lobectomy/ pneumonectomy	X	X	X	X	X	2
Coronary artery bypass graft	X	X	X	X	X	4
Cardiac valve replacement	X	X	X	X	X	4
Vascular surgery						
Femoral embolectomy	X	X	X	X	X	X
Femoro-popliteal/distal bypass	X	X	X	X	X	X
Femoro/axillo-femoral bypass	X	X	X	X	X	X
Aortoiliac/bifemoral bypass	X	X	X	X	X	2
Elective repair of aortic aneurysm	X	X	X	X	X	4
Repair of ruptured aortic aneurysm	X	X	X	X	X	6
Carotid endarterectomy	X	X	X	X	X	X
Percutaneous angioplasty	X	X	X	X	X	X
Amputation of the leg	X	X	X	X	X	X
Orthopaedic operations						
Operations for shoulder dislocation	X	X	X	X	X	X
Open reduction/fixation of arm fractures	X	X	X	X	X	
Amputations of the arm	X	X	X	X	X	
Surgery for fractured neck of femur	X	X	X	X	X	X
Total hip replacement	X	X	X	X	X	2
Internal fixation of fractured femur	X	X	X	X	X	X
Total knee replacement	X	X	X	X	X	X
Open fixation of leg fractures	X	X	X	X	X	X
Arthroscopic procedures	X	X	X	X	X	
Laminectomy	X	X	X	X	X	X

ABGs	X-ray	ITU	Bowel prep	Antibiotics	Mark site	Comments
						Results of cytology, USS and mammogram
						Results of cytology, USS and mammogram
						Exclude local recurrence
X		X	X	X		Barium swallow, oesophagoscopy and biopsies
X		X	X	X		Barium swallow, oesophagoscopy and biopsies
		X	X	X		Neomycin and lactulose for encephalopathy
X	X	X		X		
X	X	X		X		Bronchoscopy and mediastinoscopy, biopsies
X		X		X		Coronary angiograms
X		X		X		Echocardiography and radiology
					X	Full anticoagulation if diagnosis suspected
				X	X	Angiography and Doppler ankle pressures
				X	X	Angiography and Doppler ankle pressures
		X		X		Angiography and Doppler ankle pressures
X		X		X		USS/CT of aneurysm, Doppler ankle pressures
X		X		X		Resuscitate on way to theatre
X		X			X	Angiograms, Doppler studies
					X	Doppler ankle pressure studies
X				X	X	
					X	
				X	X	Radiology, check peripheral pulses
					X	
X	X			X	X	Radiology
	?X			X	X	Radiology
				X	X	Radiology
				X	X	Radiology
	X			X	X	Radiology and check peripheral pulses
					X	Radiology
						Results of CT/MRI, document neurology

Table 3.1 (contd)
Operation planner for common major operations

Operation	FBC	SMAC	CXR	ECG	Clotting	G&S/XM	
Orthopaedic operations (contd)							
Spinal fusion	X	X	X	X	X		4
Surgery for osteomyelitis	X	X	X	X	X	X	
Head, neck and endocrine							
Block dissection of the neck	X	X	X	X	X		2
Parotidectomy	X	X	X	X	X		
Excision of branchial cyst	X	X	X	X	X		
Thyroidectomy	X	X	X	X	X	X	
Parathyroidectomy	X	X	X	X	X	X	
Excision of thyroglossal cyst	X	X	X	X	X		
Adrenalectomy	X	X	X	X	X		2
Tracheostomy	X	X	X	X	X		
Laryngectomy	X	X	X	X	X		4
Gastric operations							
Gastrostomy	X	X	X	X			
Vagotomy (all types)	X	X	X	X			
Pyloric stenosis (child)	X	X				X	
Pyloric stenosis (adult)	X	X	X	X		X	
Partial gastrectomy	X	X	X	X			2
Total gastrectomy	X	X	X	X	X		2
Thoracoabdominal gastrectomy	X	X	X	X	X		4
Hellers operation	X	X	X	X		X	
Surgery for bleeding DU/GU	X	X	X	X	X		4
Repair of hiatus hernia	X	X	X	X		X	
Hepatobiliary operations							
Cholecystectomy (all types)	X	X	X	X	X	X	
Exploration of the CBD	X	X	X	X	X	X	
Choledochoduodenostomy	X	X	X	X	X	X	
Hepaticjejunostomy	X	X	X	X	X		4
Hepatectomy (right/left)	X	X	X	X	X		6
Pancreatoduodenectomy (Whipple)	X	X	X	X	X		4
Distal pancreatectomy	X	X	X	X	X		2
Splenectomy	X	X	X	X	X		platelets+2
Shunt for portal hypertension	X	X	X	X	X		4
Drainage of pseudocyst	X	X	X	X	X		2

ABGs	X-ray	ITU	Bowel prep	Antibiotics	Mark site	Comments
X	X	X		X		Radiology, document neurology
				X		Radiology, results of microbiology
				X	X	Results of cytology, EUA and biopsies
					X	Sialogram, USS/CT, check 7th nerve
					X	Cytology and USS
						USS/thyroid scan, thyroid function, recurrent nerve
						Serum Ca^{2+}, PTH, USS/CT, check vocal cords
	?X					USS/thyroid scan
					X	Adrenal function tests, USS/CT, angiogram, MIBG
	X					
X	X			X		EUA and biopsy results
						Results of gastric secretion studies
X						Correct dehydration and acid-base imbalance
X				X		Correct dehydration and acid-base imbalance
				X		Barium radiology and biopsy results
X		?X		X		Barium radiology and biopsy results
X		X		X		Barium radiology and biopsy results
						Barium swallow and oesophageal manometry
X		?X		X		Results of preoperative endoscopy
						Results of radiology and endoscopy
	X			X		USS report
	X			X		Radiology and vitamin K
	X			X		Radiology and vitamin K
	X	?X		X		Radiology and vitamin K
X	?X	X		X		Results of CT and angiography
	X			X		CT, angiography and vitamin K
		?X		X		Results of CT
		?X		X		Pneumococcus vaccination
X		X		X		Oral neomycin and lactulose for encephalopathy
	?X			X		Results of USS/CT

Table 3.1 (*contd*)
Operation planner for common major operations

Operation	FBC	SMAC	CXR	ECG	Clotting	G&S/XM	
Small and large bowel							
Laparotomy for intestinal obstruction	X	X	X	X			2
Laparotomy for Crohn's disease	X	X	X	X	X		2
Appendicectomy	X	X	X	X			
Right hemicolectomy	X	X	X	X		X	
Left hemicolectomy	X	X	X	X		X	
Sigmoid colectomy	X	X	X	X		X	
Hartmann procedure	X	X	X	X		X	
Subtotal colectomy	X	X	X	X			2
Colectomy for fulminent colitis	X	X	X	X	X		4
Anterior resection of the rectum	X	X	X	X			2
Abdominoperineal resection of rectum	X	X	X	X			3
Repair of rectal prolapse	X	X	X	X		X	
Urology (always send MSSU for MC&S)							
Endoscopic resection of bladder tumour	X	X	X	X	X	X	
TURP	X	X	X	X	X	X	
Simple nephrectomy	X	X	X	X	X	X	
Radical nephrectomy	X	X	X	X	X		3
Pyelo- or uretero-lithotomy	X	X	X	X	X	X	
Nephroureterectomy	X	X	X	X	X		2
Pyeloplasty	X	X	X	X	X	X	
Partial cystectomy	X	X	X	X	X	X	
Radical cystectomy	X	X	X	X	X		6
Urinary diversion (ileal conduit)	X	X	X	X	X	X	
Ureteric reimplantation	X	X	X	X	X	X	
Kidney transplantation	X	X	X	X	X	X	
Repair of vesicovaginal/rectal fistula	X	X	X	X	X		2
Urethroplasty	X	X	X	X	X	X	

G&S/XM is group and save or units cross matched; ABGs are arterial blood gases ar
radiology; radiology means results of previous X-rays.

ABGs	X-ray	ITU	Bowel prep	Antibiotics	Mark site	Comments
X				X		Rehydrate and resuscitate
				X	X	Results of barium studies
				X		
			X	X		Results of barium studies/ colonoscopy
			X	X		Results of barium studies/ colonoscopy
			X	X		Results of barium studies/ colonoscopy
			?X	X	X	Results of barium studies/ colonoscopy
			X	X		Results of barium studies/ colonoscopy
X		X		X	X	Rehydrate and resuscitate
			X	X		Results of barium studies/ colonoscopy
			X	X	X	Results of barium studies/ colonoscopy
			X	X		Results of rectal manometry
				X		IVU and urine cytology results
				X		Bladder USS, urodynamics, PSA/acid phosphatase
			X	X	X	IVU/USS
		?X		X	X	IVU/USS/CT and angiogram
	X			X	X	X-ray on way to theatre, position of stone
				X	X	IVU/USS urine cytology and cytoscopy
				X	X	IVU and renogram
				X		Cystoscopy, biopsies, rectal USS, pelvic CT
		X	X	X	X	Cystoscopy, biopsies, rectal USS, pelvic CT
			X	X	X	
				X		
X	X			X		Blood group and tissue type
		X		X		IVU and barium enema results
				X		Results of urethroscopy and urethrogram

...iratory function tests; ITU means book an ITU bed; X-ray means intraoperative

- Bowel preparation. All major GI surgery should be preceded by preoperative bowel prep (see page 221).
- Prophylactic antibiotic cover. Essential for all major cardiothoracic, orthopaedic, GI and vascular surgery (see page 210).
- Mark the site or side of surgery. Always mark the side of any procedure that is undertaken on a structure that exists bilaterally (e.g. hernia, hand, leg). In addition, certain procedures, such as varicose vein surgery and fashioning a colostomy, need to have the site of surgery marked before the patient goes to theatre.
- DVT/PE prophylaxis. Each hospital has its own policy; however, as a general rule patients who are over 40 years or undergoing major surgery (>30 min), women on the OCP or HRT or those for whom prolonged immobilization is expected should be prescribed TED stockings and i.m. sodium heparin 5000 units b.d., beginning on the morning of surgery and continuing until the patient is mobile. Exceptions to this are patients with peripheral vascular disease, who should not be given TED stockings, orthopaedic patients, who may benefit from low-molecular-weight heparin such as Fragmin, and those already on anticoagulants.

Marking up varicose veins

This should be the job of the Surgeon who will do the operation but may be delegated to you.

- If it has been decided the patient needs a groin tie (ligation of the sapheno-femoral junction), mark the groin.
- Test the competence of the valve at the sapheno-femoral junction yourself by seeing if pressure over this point controls the varicosities. Sapheno-femoral incompetence accounts for the vast majority of varicose veins. In addition, the patient may have been on the waiting list for some considerable time since he/she was originally seen and the nature of the necessary surgery determined. The veins may have become significantly worse over this period.
- Mark out all the varicose tributaries with a *permanent* marker pen (Fig. 3.1). Do not use anything that is water or alcohol soluble as it will wash out when the leg is prepped for surgery. Your reference will go down the drain with the surgical spirit!

The short saphenous vein runs from behind the lateral malleolus to enter the popliteal vein lateral to the midline at the back of the knee (Fig. 3.1a). True short saphenous varicosities are unusual. Pay specific attention to the course of the long saphenous vein that runs from anterior to the medial malleolus directly to the femoral vein at the groin (Fig. 3.1b).

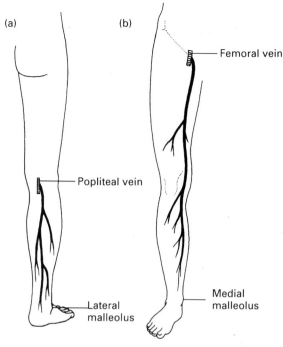

Fig. 3.1 Marking varicose veins. Route of (a) short saphenous vein and (b) long saphenous vein.

Siting an end colostomy/ileostomy

These procedures are best undertaken with the direct collaboration of the Stoma Therapist. Essentially they are the same procedure, except that an ileostomy is sited in the right iliac fossa and an end colostomy is sited in the left iliac fossa.

- With the patient standing, mark the mid-point between the umbilicus and the anterior superior iliac spine (Fig. 3.2a).
- Repeat the exercise with the patient seated (Fig. 3.2b) and then lying flat.
- Note any obvious skin creases or scars adjacent to or within these marks.
- The final position is a compromise between the three positions (which may all be the same), but away from any skin creases and scars.
- Place a stoma bag over the site and get the patient to dress in normal attire. Make sure that the site does not interfere with clothing, particularly belts and tight-fitting skirts.

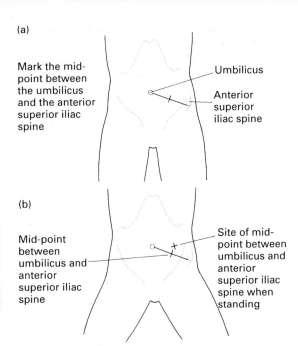

(a)

Mark the mid-point between the umbilicus and the anterior superior iliac spine

Umbilicus

Anterior superior iliac spine

(b)

Mid-point between umbilicus and anterior superior iliac spine

Site of mid-point between umbilicus and anterior superior iliac spine when standing

Fig. 3.2 Siting an end colostomy (left iliac fossa) or ileostomy (right iliac fossa). (a) With the patient standing; (b) with the patient seated.

Putting together the operating list

This may fall to you, or it may be the responsibility of some other member of the team. There are one or two basic rules about the order of any operating list.

Patients who come at the *front* of the list are:

- Children
- Diabetics
- Major cases requiring a postoperative ITU bed.

Patients who go at the *end* of the list are:

- Colorectal cases, in particular anal procedures
- Drainage of abscesses
- Patients who are, or potentially are, biohazards (hepatitis, HIV positive or AIDS).

The list will need to be with the operating theatre by the middle of the afternoon of the day before. Any subsequent changes must be made in writing on *all copies* of the list by a medically qualified member of the surgeon's team. This will avoid any confusion over the wrong patient being sent for, or receiving, the wrong operation.

The night before the list

Contact the Anaesthetist who is going to give the anaesthetics to the patients on your list. Explain the order of the list and any specific medical problems of the patients on the list. This will preclude any last minute ranting and raving by the Anaesthetic Department at 8.00 am the next day about lack of consultation over patients appearing on the list with bizarre tropical disorders or down-to-earth problems such as diabetes. For further advice on surviving the Anaesthetist, see page 80.

The day of the list

Ensure that the case notes are available and are up to date. Assemble *all* your patients' relevant investigations with the case notes. Make sure that all the patients' X-rays are present. Any omissions here are entirely your fault; it is no-one else's responsibility to collect these items together and deliver them to the operating theatre.

Postoperative care

1. Read your patients' operation notes and postoperative care instructions from both the Surgeon and the Anaesthetist.
2. Carefully examine the postoperative prescriptions for fluids, analgesia, antibiotics and any other drug that has been commenced during or at the end of surgery.
3. Find out what specimens (histological, cytological and microbiological) from your patients were sent from the operating room to the laboratory.
4. Familiarize yourself with the various tubes and drains now attached to your patients.

Outside of intensive care, postoperative measurements include the following.

Minor surgery

- 4-hourly pulse and blood pressure.

Major surgery

- Hourly pulse and blood pressure (CVP if a line is in place – see page 179)
- Hourly urine output (if a catheter is in place)
- 4-hourly nasogastric aspirate
- 24-hourly charting of drain output.

Postoperative investigations

After *minor surgery*, such as inguinal hernia repair, no investigations are necessary.

After *major surgery*, measure the following:

- FBC on the first day

- Daily electrolytes until drinking normally
- Electrolyte measurements of high output effluents, e.g. nasogastric aspirate (see page 173)
- Daily CXR after thoracic procedures, until the chest drains are removed
- Histology of resected specimens
- Microbiology of cultures sent from the operating room and review the patient's antibiotic regimen accordingly.

EMERGENCY SURGERY

As patients are admitted from A&E with problems that require emergency surgery the basic ground rules are the same as for elective admission. The differences are firstly that such patients are not being worked-up for a routine elective list and, secondly, the patient may require some degree of resuscitation prior to surgery (see page 51). However, it is your responsibility, and no-one else's, to ensure that all the relevant details of investigation, resuscitation and preoperative treatment arrive with your patient in the operating room.

SURVIVING THE ANAESTHETIST

Most Anaesthetists are relatively benign and understanding; however, they do not like to be seen as the surgeon's lackey or as someone who wishes to avoid patient contact. Anaesthetists do not work in firms like other hospital clinicians. However, your Consultant will probably work regularly with the same Consultant Anaesthetist, and he/she will usually be assisted by the same Junior Anaesthetist for some period of time. Get to know these particular Anaesthetists, particularly their foibles and peculiarities, especially with regard to letting them know about the proposed operating list. This is particularly the case with difficult anaesthetic problems.

Preoperative investigations: which tests and why

A major source of strife for House Surgeons is the uncertainty over which preoperative investigations will be required by which Anaesthetist for each patient. These are summarized above (see pages 70–75). Most anaesthetists will have firm views on which tests are essential and which are optional – unfortunately, many of these opinions will be at variance with other Anaesthetists. On many occasions, strict adherence to these policies is wasteful both financially and also of your time. Get to know what your particular Anaesthetist likes in the preoperative work-up. The addition of a small amount of common sense and medical knowledge will allow you to develop a rational approach to these investigations which will keep your

Consultant and his/her Anaesthetist happy and off your back and keep form-filling to a minimum.

For the best chance of a successful outcome to surgery, it is important that the patient arrives in theatre in optimal condition. This state may be compromised by the condition requiring surgery, or by co-existing disease. All investigations must be justified by an expectation that the result could be abnormal. Preoperative investigations are not a screening exercise for the general population.

The anaesthetic decision of whether a patient is fit for a general anaesthetic is based on history, examination and investigations. The major anaesthetic concern is with the *cardiovascular* and *respiratory* systems. If an abnormality is detected and is correctable, then the decision to delay surgery until such correction is made jointly between the Surgeon and the Anaesthetist.

Cardiovascular system (see also page 48)

Any necessary investigations are usually suggested by the history and examination. An ECG will diagnose ischaemic heart disease and dysrhythmias. The incidence of 'silent ischaemia' is significant and ischaemic heart disease is associated with many other pathological conditions (cerebrovascular disease, hypertension, diabetes, etc.). A preoperative ECG on all patients over the age of 50 is recommended. Under the age of 50, an ECG should be carried out in the following conditions:

- History of chest pains, palpitations, shortness of breath on exertion, syncope (sudden fainting)
- Hypertension (systolic >160 mmHg, diastolic >100 mmHg)
- History of heart disease
- Strong family history of heart disease
- Heavy smoker (>25 cigarettes/day).

Respiratory system (see also page 54)

Most information regarding the respiratory system comes from the history. If these symptoms are significant it is important to determine if they can be improved before surgery. Shortness of breath is really a question of degree and tolerance. If someone who complains of dyspnoea on exertion can walk half a mile uphill to the pub, then as a rule they are not hovering on the brink of respiratory failure. If, however, walking across the room leaves them gasping for air, they will need to be handled and treated very carefully indeed. If a patient is normally fit but has a cough or cold, it is customary to postpone surgery until they are better. This is because general anaesthesia causes some atelectasis (alveolar collapse), which in the presence of co-existing upper airway infection may lead to bronchopneumonia. The most common causes of chronic shortness of breath on exertion are COPD (chronic bronchitis and emphysema), asthma and heart failure. These should be apparent from the history and clinical examination. If any of these factors concern you, contact the Anaesthetist immediately. Lower airway obstruction produces a wheeze which can be reversed, at least in part, by bronchodilators. Inspiratory wheeze (stridor) is a serious sign, indicating upper airway obstruction. Exclude an obstructing tumour or, more rarely, a foreign body.

Concurrent upper respiratory tract infection is only a relative contraindication in emergency surgery. If the surgical condition is life-threatening then it cannot be deferred. In this situation it is necessary to optimize the perioperative state using antibiotics, oxygen, bronchodilators and chest physiotherapy. These decisions, particularly in the emergency situation, should be made at Consultant level.

Routine chest X-ray   This is often a pointless exercise. It is only of value if there is a history of previous pulmonary disease or physical signs indicate significant pathology (bronchial breathing suggesting lobar consolidation; haemoptysis and stridor suggesting a bronchogenic carcinoma).

Pulmonary function tests   Provide valuable points of reference and should be requested for patients who have significant respiratory impairment. The most important values are:

- FEV_1 (forced expiratory volume in 1 s) is normally 4 litres – <50% of predicted value indicates a serious degree of airway obstruction or restriction.
- FVC (forced vital capacity) is normally 5 litres.
- The ratio FEV_1/FVC will allow differentiation between an obstructive and a restrictive pattern of airway disease. FEV_1/FVC <70% indicates an obstructive pattern. The effect of bronchodilators on obstruction may be assessed; the obstruction may be partially reversible. A restrictive airway disease may give more problems for the anaesthetist (e.g. cystic fibrosis, gross kyphoscoliosis). ABG estimation gives an accurate indication of the efficiency of alveolar gas exchange, and the degree of derangement (if existing) to the central control of respiration. The inspired oxygen concentration should always be noted, otherwise the PaO_2 value is meaningless.

Blood tests

Full blood count   Reduction in blood haemoglobin concentration results in reduced blood oxygen-carrying capacity. Elevated haemoglobin concentration, usually associated with increased numbers of erythrocytes, is associated with increased blood viscosity, and sludging of capillary blood flow. Optimal delivery of oxygen to tissues occurs at a happy medium between anaemia and polycythaemia.

Maximum (optimal) tissue oxygen delivery occurs at a haematocrit of 0.3 (30% of the blood volume is occupied by erythrocytes), corresponding to a haemoglobin concentration of 10 g/dl. Haemoglobin concentrations below this are not a contraindication to elective surgery or an indication for pre-operative transfusion. Only if the serum haemoglobin is <8 g/dl should serious thought be given to delaying surgery and consideration of blood transfusion. In addition there are many chronic causes of low serum haemoglobin concentration (sickle cell, thalassaemia, etc.) and it may well be appropriate to operate on a patient with such a low serum haemoglobin. If you find your patient to be anaemic and this is associated with the condition warranting surgical intervention, liaise with the Anaesthetist regarding the necessity for transfusion. If the patient is anaemic and this is totally unexpected (e.g. a patient undergoing elective cholecystectomy for gallstones), then the anaemia should be investigated and managed as a priority over the elective surgery. *Always* let the Anaesthetist know in good time that they are to anaesthetize an anaemic patient.

When should the haemoglobin always be measured?

- Prior to major surgery, particularly where blood loss may be significant. As a rule of thumb, a fall of 1 g/dl in haemoglobin concentration is equivalent to the loss of 1 unit of blood.

- If anaemia is suspected (history of GI bleeding, heavy periods, chronic renal failure, rheumatoid arthritis, cancer, sickle cell disease).

- If a bleeding tendency is suspected (anticoagulant therapy, liver disease, thrombocytopenia). In these cases the request for an FBC must be accompanied by a request for a clotting profile. Abnormalities in clotting such as a defect in the clotting pathway or inadequate platelets (number or function) should be discussed with both the Anaesthetist and the Haematologist. Arrangements can then be made to have the necessary factors (platelets or fresh frozen plasma) available to cover the proposed surgery.

Sickle cell test   The presence of an abnormal variant of the haemoglobin molecule, haemoglobin S (HbS), is detected by a simple laboratory investigation called the 'Sickledex' test. This test does not distinguish between homozygous (all the haemoglobin in the red cell is HbS) or heterozygous (half the haemoglobin in the red cell is HbS) state.

Patients homozygous for HbS suffer from classical sickle cell disease with all its well-described manifestations. The major problem with regard to anaesthesia is that hypoxia or dehydration associated with the stress of surgery and general anaesthesia may precipitate sickling of the red cells and a sickle crisis. Most heterozygous patients are termed sickle trait. This trait is very common in people from areas where malaria is endemic, since sickle trait confers some resistance to the disease. HbS has been identified in *all* non-Caucasian people, with the exception of Chinese and Japanese. Therefore a 'Sickledex' test is mandatory in all these cases prior to general anaesthesia. A positive 'Sickledex' test should automatically lead to haemoglobin electrophoresis to determine whether the patient is homozygous or heterozygous.

Electrolytes Abnormal serum potassium frightens Anaesthetists. Hyper- or hypokalaemia predisposes to cardiac arrhythmias and reduction in myocardial contractility (see p. 226).

Serum sodium is rarely abnormal unless there is a serious underlying metabolic disturbance (severe dehydration or water overload, Addison's disease, Conn's syndrome).

Serum urea is an indicator of degree of hydration (in patients with normal renal function) and in conjunction with serum creatinine, a measure of renal function if there is established kidney disease.

Serum glucose Fasting serum glucose should be measured preoperatively in all diabetic patients prior to elective surgery under general anaesthesia, regardless of the severity of their diabetes and the nature of the surgery. All patients admitted to the surgical ward should have their urine routinely examined for the presence of glucose. If diabetes is suspected, then elective surgery should be deferred until this is sorted out.

Summary

Investigations required for:

Minor surgery

- Fit and well, >50 years – ECG, if not done in the preceding 6 months + CXR + U & E + FBC

Intermediate surgery (e.g. varicose veins, haemorrhoidectomy)

- Fit and well, >50 years – Hb + ECG, if not done in the preceding 6 months + CXR + U & E

Major surgery (e.g. laparotomy, total hip replacement)

- Fit and well, >50 years – Hb + group and save of serum/ appropriate cross-match + CXR + U & E
- Fit and well, >50 years – Hb, group and save/cross-match, ECG + CXR + U & E

Remember: *If in doubt, consult the Anaesthetist*

4

The postoperative period ('Doctor, Doctor!')

85

As a House Surgeon you will frequently be telephoned in the middle of the night when patients develop problems in the post-operative period. Nobody likes being telephoned at 3 am, but it is essential to develop a logical method of investigating common postoperative problems. Before putting the phone down make sure you know the patient's age, what surgery they've had and what their basic observations are (if these have not been done, politely ask for them to be available on your arrival). As you trudge through the cold air from your bed to the surgical ward, *think* about the presenting complaint and all of its possible causes. A simple example of this is a patient who has stopped passing urine. Remember that the catheter may be blocked. Think about potential causes of hypotension in the post-operative period (sepsis, haemorrhage). Make a mental note of the simple investigations and procedures that you might reasonably be expected to perform in order to solve the patient's problems.

Having arrived *on the ward*, carefully take a history from and examine the patient. Whilst doing this, keep in mind the common causes of anuria (or whatever the patient's complaint might be). Next, instigate any simple *investigations* that might be appropriate and decide whether someone more senior needs to be involved in this particular postoperative complication.

Any postoperative complication heralded by a phone call at 3 am should be dealt with in this simple fashion:

1. Ask for the patient's age, observations and recent surgical history before putting down the phone.
2. Think about the patient and complication whilst walking to the ward.
3. Take a history and examine the patient carefully on arrival on the ward.
4. Instigate simple investigations and decide whether someone more senior is needed to deal with the problem.
5. Instigate simple treatment and be sure to review the progress of your treatment, either later that night or the next morning.

Another important principle when dealing with such emergencies is to make sure you personally see all the results of the investigations you have ordered. It is pointless to order a CXR and then leave the ward without carefully looking at it! You may feel a patient is sufficiently ill to call a more senior colleague before all your investigations are completed but as a rule it is helpful to have a concise summary of your clinical findings and some simple investigations when you phone for a second opinion on your patient.

If the patient to whom you are called is not normally under your care, make sure you both read the recent notes carefully and ask the nurses on the ward for any salient details about the person. In days of increasing cross-cover you may frequently be asked to sort out quite complex problems in patients totally unknown to you.

HYPOTENSION

You will *often* be called because a patient has a low blood pressure.

Think

The most common causes of postoperative hypotension are:

- Haemorrhage
- Sepsis
- Cardiac.

On the ward

1. If you are familiar with the patient go straight to him/her, take a history and do an examination. If not, make sure you get hold of the notes to review the operative procedure and postoperative progress and then go and see the patient with the notes.
2. Is the patient well or distressed? It is not unheard of to be called to see a patient who is sound asleep with no obvious sign of disease, but who happens to have a blood pressure of 85/50 and a pulse of 60. Clearly, such a patient is not in need of emergency resuscitation unless there has been some recent change in his/her haemodynamic status, or evidence of severe haemorrhage and sepsis.
3. Examine the patient for signs of haemorrhage. This may be obvious, as in the case of haematemesis and melaena. Be sure to check the operative drains and wound areas in case of haematoma.
4. Check for signs of sepsis; in particular, note any productive cough or urinary symptoms as well as any cellulitis.
5. Make sure you examine the pulse, blood pressure and temperature chart, noting particularly any change in haemodynamic stability and any previous similar episodes.

Investigations

Haemorrhage

1. Make sure the patient has good intravenous access. Use at least a green intravenous canula (21 gauge) and turn up the rate of flow of the intravenous fluid attached to the drip (as long as there is not a large amount of potassium in the bag) (see page 170)
2. Once you are happy with intravenous access, take blood for FBC, U & E, clotting screen and cross-match. Undertake these investigations as an emergency and make sure that you chase the results and write them down in the notes before returning to bed.
3. In cases of haemorrhage, you will want to contact your next on-call for advice; this is particularly the case when

Management of postoperative hypotension

Postoperative hypotension
|
Resuscitate
– airway
– breathing
– circulation (colloid)
|
Establish cause
|
CVP

Low
|
Continue colloid infusion
|
? Fluid depletion/ inadequate replenishment
– replace
? Bleeding
– revealed
– concealed
|
Return to operating room

Normal
|
? Septic
– blood cultures
– urine cultures
– drain fluid
– sputum cultures
– blood gases
– clotting
– FBC

High
|
? Cardiac
– ECG
– cardiac enzymes
|
? MI
? Fluid overload
– call duty medical team

Wound sepsis

Laparotomy (GI/urology)

Other wounds

Antibiotics for Gram negative organisms and anaerobes

Respiratory sepsis
– oxygen
– physiotherapy
– antibiotics for Gram positive organisms

Urinary sepsis

Abdominal sepsis (inc. biliary sepsis)

Antibiotics for Gram negative organisms and anaerobes

Elective
– antibiotics for Gram positive organisms

Trauma
– antibiotics for Gram positive and negative organisms and anaerobes; penicillin for Clostridia

the haemorrhage has been large enough to disturb the patient's haemodynamic stability.
4. A rapid assessment of the grade of shock is necessary and will help management (Table 4.1).

Sepsis

1. Make sure you have good intravenous access with at least a green intravenous canula (21 gauge).
2. Take blood for FBC, U & E and blood cultures.
3. Take cultures from sputum, urine or wound edge as appropriate.
4. Increase rate of intravenous infusions and, in the absence of any organisms, start appropriate broad-spectrum antibiotics (cefuroxime 750 mg t.d.s., metronidazole 400 mg b.d. are a common choice after bowel surgery).
5. If you are at all concerned about the patient, contact your next on-call to discuss their management.
6. Write the results of your investigations in the notes and institute half-hourly observations on the patient to chart progress.

TACHYCARDIA

Think
A tachycardia may be due to:

- Something simple like inadequate analgesia
- cardiac arrhythmia
- Hypovolaemia
- Sepsis

On the ward

1. Assess the patient (are they in pain or not?).
2. Does the patient have symptoms associated with the tachycardia (shortness of breath, palpitations or chest pain)?
3. Examine the patient and check the pulse, blood pressure and temperature. Also listen to heart sounds and examine for a raised JVP.
4. Check the drug kardex and see how much analgesia has been given and how recently. Also make a note of any other cardiovascular medication that the patient was taking preoperatively.

Investigations

- If the patient has a *sinus tachycardia* which seems to be related to undue postoperative pain, no investigations are necessary and a dose of analgesia may solve the problem.

Table 4.1
Classification of hypovolaemic shock according to blood losses (in a 70 kg man)

	Class 1	Class 2	Class 3	Class 4
Blood loss (ml)	up to 750	750–1500	1500–2000	>2000
Pulse rate	<100	100–120	120–140	>140
Blood pressure				
systolic	Normal	Normal	Reduced	Very low
diastolic	Normal	Raised	Reduced	Very low
Urinary flow rate (ml/h)	>30	20–30	10–20	<10
Respiratory rate	14–20	20–30	30–40	>40
Mental state	Alert	Anxious/aggressive	Anxious/drowsy	Drowsy/unconscious
Skin colour	Normal	Pale	Pale	Pale/cold
Fluid replacement	Crystalloid	Crystalloid	Crystalloid and blood	Crystalloid and blood

A haemorrhage of up to 1.5 litres will still give a normal systolic blood pressure. A careful clinical examination will give an estimation of the blood losses and initial fluid requirement. The patient's response to initial resuscitation is the key to subsequent therapy.

- If the patient's *pulse* is in any way abnormal, or there is a suspicion of underlying myocardial disease, an ECG and CXR must be performed. It is also often desirable to take blood for FBC, U & E and cardiac enzymes.
- If the tachycardia is associated with *hypotension*, then management should follow as for hypotension (see page 88).

ANURIA/OLIGURIA

The phone call reporting a reduced or absent urine output in a postoperative patient must be one of the most common for a House Surgeon, and it is important to deal in a logical and sequential manner with this problem (see also page 63).

Think
Oliguria is often considered to be the passage of <30 ml of urine per hour. This is a good general guide but it should be remembered that in small people (<60 kg) an output of 15–20 ml/h may be perfectly acceptable as long as they are producing urine with an osmolality greater than serum and are clinically well hydrated.

1. Has the patient got a urinary catheter in place or not?
2. Reduced urine output may be due to prerenal, renal or postrenal causes.

In the surgical patient with a urinary catheter, the most common postrenal cause is a blocked catheter. In addition, postoperative patients have all had some degree of hypotension during and after surgery and are more prone to sepsis. Both hypotension and sepsis will act to reduce urine output by prerenal and renal mechanisms. Assess carefully your patient's haemodynamic status when you get to the ward.

On the ward
1. Check for a history of previous renal impairment.
2. Make sure the patient is not on any potentially nephrotoxic drugs (e.g. aminoglycosides).
3. *In the patient without a catheter*, look particularly for evidence of an enlarged bladder. If they appear to be in urinary retention, place a catheter (see page 174).
4. *In the patient with a catheter* already in place do not start tugging on the patient's catheter straight away. Be sure to talk to the patient, assess their clinical state, giving particular heed to any signs of hypotension or sepsis and explain to him/her why you are about to fiddle with their catheter. The patient may be unaware of his/her oliguria and will not welcome a sudden nocturnal tug on their catheter.

5. Examine for signs of:
   – Hypotension (renal perfusion)
   – Renal bruits (renal vascular disease)
   – Femoral pulses (especially after aneurysm surgery)
   – JVP/CVP if in situ/lung bases/oedema (fluid balance)
   – DVT (possible renal vein thrombosis).
6. Examine the fluid balance chart and, in particular, note the hourly urine output over the previous 24 h.
7. Examine the catheter bag and, as a first line of investigation, flush the catheter. This is undertaken with a 50 ml bladder syringe. Fill this with 30 ml of sterile saline, which is then gently instilled into the bladder. Withdraw with the syringe, noting whether >30 ml is removed from the bladder. If no more than a total of 30 ml returns, then it is unlikely that the catheter was blocked and further investigations will be necessary.

Investigations

1. Ensure good venous access and take blood for FBC and U & E.
2. If there is doubt about the cause of anuria, check the osmolality of the most recent catheter specimen. Urine >300 mOsm/kg suggests that the kidney is concentrating urine (functioning normally), and intravenous fluids may resolve the anuria/oliguria. An osmolality of 300 mOsm/kg or less, or thereabouts, suggests that the kidney has failed to concentrate urine and the patient is in renal failure.
3. If the patient appears to have a *negative fluid balance* and there are no clinical signs of fluid overload (raised JVP, fine crepitations at the chest bases, dependent oedema – usually sacral in the recumbent patient), then institute a 500 ml fluid challenge. To do this, infuse 500 ml of fluid over 60 min. If dehydration was the sole cause of anuria, urinary output will often pick up at this point.
4. If the patient appears to have a *positive fluid balance* and does not appear dehydrated, a fluid challenge may still be employed but with some caution.
5. Do *not* simply infuse 20 mg frusemide i.v. in the hope of inducing a short-term diuresis so you can return to bed for 2 or 3 h more sleep. If the patient is dehydrated and needs more volume to increase urine output, such a procedure will simply dehydrate them further. If the patient on the other hand is in established renal failure, such a procedure will simply cause a short-term diuresis and may further damage the failing kidney as frusemide is a loop diuretic which also acts as a tubular poison and can be nephrotoxic in the failing kidney.
6. If clearing any blockage in the catheter, or administering fluid challenge, does nothing to improve urinary output, organize the insertion of a central line. An emergency US

scan of kidneys and bladder will confirm a renal or postrenal cause and the position of the catheter, if in doubt. The role of renal doses of dopamine (1–5 μg/kg) is not totally clear but may be considered. However, it would be wise to discuss the case with your immediate senior before doing this.

CONFUSION

Think

Many an elderly patient has tried to leave hospital in the 24 h after an operation, claiming they are about to be kidnapped by the Martians or the hospital is about to be sent into outer space. These may not seem unreasonable assertions at 3 am, but it is important as you walk over to the ward to go through simple biochemical causes of confusional states, in order that you may address these in the postoperative patient.

Confusion may be caused by:

- Hypoxia (most common)
- Pre-existing disease (psychiatric, metabolic, liver, renal, etc.)
- Withdrawal states (alcohol, drugs and toxins)
- Current drug therapy (amphetamines, anticholinergics, sedatives, opiates, etc.)
- Fever (per se)
- Sepsis
- Metabolic: electrolyte/glucose disturbance
- Fluids: overload or dehydration
- CNS (CVA, infection), CVS (MI, CCF, hypotension).

On the ward

Try to avoid confrontation with the patient if at all possible. History is often unhelpful, but examination may reveal a septic focus or signs of hypoxia.

Investigations

- If at all possible, venous blood should be taken for FBC, U & E, amylase and glucose.
- It may also be helpful to obtain ABGs if there is any suspicion of hypoxia. This is particularly common in patients with pre-existing lung disease who have had abdominal or thoracic operations, thus further reducing their respiratory capacity.
- If sepsis is suspected, check blood cultures, urine and sputum as well as a routine CXR.

Management

- Correction of obvious *electrolyte disturbance* such as hypo- or hyperglycaemia may reverse the confusional state.

- Correction of *hypoxia* by 35% oxygen into a mask or nasal cannula will often reverse a confusional state. In the absence of hypoxia it is still appropriate to administer oxygen as a simple treatment which can do no harm and may certainly improve the patient's condition.
- *Sepsis* should be managed as discussed under hypotension (see page 88) and in Useful Drugs (see page 210)
- It may be necessary to use major tranquillizers such as chlorpromazine 25 mg i.v./i.m., haloperidol 5 mg i.v./i.m. or chlormethiazole 250–500 mg (5–10 ml) orally. It is preferable to try and avoid widescale use of these on an empirical basis, although it is accepted that these are often necessary to prevent the patient removing all surgical drains and intravenous cannulae and leaving hospital.

SHORTNESS OF BREATH

Think
The major causes of shortness of breath in the postoperative patient are:

- Pulmonary infection
- Aspiration pneumonia
- Pulmonary oedema
- Bronchospasm
- Pulmonary embolus
- pneumothorax.

As you walk over to the ward think whether the patient has had any preoperative pulmonary disease. Also think whether the patient is particularly at risk of pulmonary embolus and always consider this in your differential diagnosis of shortness of breath.

On the ward

1. Take a history from the patient; in particular, ascertain whether the shortness of breath is of gradual onset or sudden. Sudden-onset shortness of breath is more likely to be a pulmonary embolus or pneumothorax. It may also be due to pulmonary oedema precipitated by either overtransfusion or an MI. This may often be silent in the elderly and in the postoperative patient.
2. Examine the patient carefully:
   - Look for signs of sepsis (pyrexia, productive cough, coarse crepitations in the chest)
   - Look for signs of fluid overload (raised JVP, fine crepitations in the chest, dependent oedema)
   - Listen for signs of bronchospasm (wheeze)
   - Check both calves and thighs for evidence of DVT

    – Look for signs of pneumothorax (hyperresonance on percussion, decreased breath sounds).

Investigations
Investigations are crucial:

- FBC, U & E
- CXR
- ECG
- ABGs.

Management

Chest infection

1. Having taken sputum for culture and possibly blood for culture, if your patient is systemically unwell, institute antibiotic treatment (ampicillin 500 mg q.d.s. i.v.).
2. Make sure the patient receives regular physiotherapy. This is as important as antibiotics in the postoperative period when a patient finds difficulty in coughing and clearing their large airways.
3. Remember to give oxygen by face mask (35%) or nasal cannulae.

Pulmonary oedema

1. Remember to turn down all intravenous fluids to the absolute minimum.
2. Sit the patient bolt upright.
3. Administer oxygen by face mask (35%).
4. Give frusemide 20–80 mg i.v. depending on the severity of the oedema and the size of the patient.
5. Consider a dose of opiate (diamorphine 2.5 mg i.v.).
6. If the patient has pulmonary oedema secondary to myocardial ischaemia or infarction, contact your next on-call for further advice on the patient's management.

Bronchospasm

1. Treat the patient with oxygen by face mask (35%) and a salbutamol nebulizer.
2. Consideration may be given to both aminophylline 250 mg i.v. and steroids; however, it should be remembered that aminophylline takes approximately 1 h to start acting and steroids 12 h.
3. If you are concerned that bronchospasm is not responding to your empirical treatment with salbutamol nebulizer, contact your next on-call.

Pulmonary embolus

It may be difficult to confirm your diagnosis beyond reasonable doubt without recourse to a ventilation/perfusion scintiscan. However, in a patient who has evidence of DVT and ECG changes suggestive of right heart strain (S1Q3T3), it may well be reasonable to give a bolus dose of 5000 U of heparin followed by an intravenous infusion of heparin at 1000 U/h. If this line of management is adopted, it is still wise to get a ventilation/perfusion scan the next morning to confirm beyond reasonable doubt the presence of a pulmonary embolus as this will make the decision about long-term anticoagulation of the patient easier.

Pneumothorax

The urgency of treatment will depend upon whether the pneumothorax is under tension or not. A tension pneumothorax is a life-threatening event, and if you are unsure how to proceed and the patient appears to be deteriorating, simply place a large-bore needle in the second intercostal space in the midclavicular line of the affected hemithorax. The patient will need a formal chest drain for both simple and tension pneumothorax.

CHEST PAIN

Think

There are three common causes of chest pain in the postoperative period:

- Myocardial ischaemia
- pulmonary sepsis
- pulmonary embolus.

As you walk over to the ward, remember that many patients in the postoperative period find it difficult to take a deep breath, but resolve to examine the patient whilst taking a deep breath as pleuritic chest pain is best demonstrated in this setting.

On the ward

1. Take a careful history from the patient eliciting the character of the pain. You may be surprised to discover that they in fact have had acid reflux and heartburn and have been on longstanding antacids for this. Even in the face of such a history, it may be wise to take an ECG and cardiac enzymes as MI is often difficult to spot in the immediate postoperative period.
2. Examine the patient carefully giving particular attention to any cardiac abnormalities and any signs within the chest.

Investigations

- ECG and cardiac enzymes (if there is any doubt about the cause of the patient's chest pain)
- CXR (always).

Management

Pleuritic chest pain

Consider the use of an NSAID, such as indomethacin 50 mg t.d.s. orally or 50 mg t.d.s. p.r. NSAIDs are very effective in the treatment of pleuritic chest pain and should be used in addition to treating the underlying disorder (such as sepsis).

Myocardial infarction

Give high flow O_2 (via rebreathing mask) and ensure i.v. access. If the pain has not resolved with sublingual nitrates, give a small dose of diamorphine (2.5–5 mg i.v.) to relieve the pain and consult your next on-call urgently as regards further management of the patient. It may be that observation on the coronary care unit is in the patient's best interests.

BLEEDING FROM THE GUT

Think

GI haemorrhage is a common medical and surgical emergency (see page 142). After major surgery, it is not unusual for a patient with pre-existing peptic ulcer disease to have a GI haemorrhage. Furthermore, severe stress as experienced by patients on intensive care units often leads to multiple gastric erosions and secondary GI haemorrhage.

As you walk over to the ward remember that the first priority is to assess the patient haemodynamically, obtain good venous access and cross-match blood. The niceties of the site of GI haemorrhage can be elucidated once the patient has been made safe.

On the ward

1. Make sure a large-bore i.v. cannula (brown or grey venflon) is in place. Take blood for urgent FBC, U & E and cross-match.
2. Examine the patient, taking careful note of pulse, blood pressure and peripheral perfusion.
3. Try to make a careful estimate of the volume of haematemesis or melaena that the patient has passed. In doing so, remember that this will only be a proportion of the total amount of blood lost.
4. Take a brief history (and/or read the notes/speak to the nurses), with particular reference to previous dyspepsia, frank ulcer disease and drugs (e.g. NSAIDs, proton pump inhibitors, etc.).
5. Consideration should be given to a urinary catheter, central venous line and immediate endoscopy or laparotomy, and these are best discussed with your next on-call.

> ### Remember
>
> As a general rule, haematemesis and melaena, which have caused haemodynamic instability in a patient, will need at least 3 units of blood to redress the balance.
>
> In the case of questionable GI haemorrhage where vomit is bile-stained but not frank blood, or bowel motion appears slightly runny, but not the classical tarry melaena stool, examine the vomit or bowel motion yourself to decide whether it is blood.
>
> The use of the haemoccult test on either vomit or faeces in this situation is useless. It is highly sensitive to the presence of blood, picking up as little as 1 part per 1 000 000 and vomit or bowel motion in a postoperative patient is nearly always haemoccult positive, but rarely haematemesis and melaena. It is therefore important that you are not swayed by information suggesting that the vomit or faeces are haemoccult positive: examine them yourself.

BLEEDING FROM THE WOUND

Think

Most haemorrhage from surgical wounds will settle spontaneously. Occasionally there is a small visible vessel causing the haemorrhage and this may be underrun. Even more infrequently, haemorrhage may be due to serious underlying problems such as arterial bleeding after vascular surgery – always consider this possibility after such surgery.

Remember that the patient may have some underlying clotting deficiency. There are three broad patterns of abnormal bleeding:

- Purpura or spontaneous haemorrhage usually caused by vessel wall or platelet disorders.
- Bleeding from trauma (surgery), which is usually due to a clotting factor deficiency.
- Total haemostatic failure due to a combination of platelet and clotting factor deficiency.

On the ward

Examine the wound yourself. Carefully remove any pressure dressings so that you can inspect the wound fully. Note whether the patient's blood is clotting and whether there are any other signs of coagulopathy (excessive bruising/haemorrhage from other sites).

Investigations

Usually there is no need to investigate a patient with wound-edge bleeding but if you suspect impaired clotting as the cause of haemorrhage then it is wise to check the FBC, clotting screen and cross-match blood.

Management

- In the presence of *superficial slow ooze* from the wound edges, place a pressure dressing of gauze onto the wound, taped firmly down with a strong adhesive tape such as zinc oxide tape.
- If a *small visible vessel* from the wound edge can be identified as the cause of haemorrhage, underrun with a 2/0 non-absorbable suture and tie off the vessel. This is done by placing the stich 2–3 mm back from the skin edge, 2–3 mm away from the bleeding vessel running underneath it and coming back up through the skin 2–3 mm on the other side of the vessel. A knot is then tied which should occlude the small arterial vessel.
- If *haemorrhage* appears to be more serious call your next on-call.
- In cases of *direct arterial haemorrhage* (most common from groin incisions after arterial surgery), make sure that either you or a senior nurse maintains direct pressure over the bleeding point. It is quite possible for a patient to exsanguinate from a leaking femoral artery!

BACK ACHE

It is *unlikely* that you will be called in the middle of the night to a patient with back ache, although *expanding or leaking aortic aneurysm* and *pancreatitis* may both present pre-dominantly with back ache. Other common conditions, such as *ureteric calculi*, may also be reported to you as a patient with back ache. On the daily ward round, however, many postoperative patients have musculoskeletal aches and pains after surgery. Patients with pre-existing *osteoarthritis* may find an exacerbation of their back ache after several hours on the operating table. Similarly, operations where patients are placed in an unusual position (e.g. nephrectomy), are more likely to cause *musculoskeletal aches and pains*.

Always consider more serious causes of back ache (such as aneurysm or pancreatitis) when a patient complains, but remember that the majority will have non-life-threatening pathologies as the cause of this back ache. If back ache persists for more than a few days, plain spinal X-rays and consideration of a referral to an orthopaedic surgeon may be appropriate.

CONSTIPATION

It is *unlikely* that you will be called to see a patient in the small hours of the morning because of constipation. However, it is a common occurrence after any form of surgery. A combination of reduced oral intake and postoperative opiates may produce quite severe constipation, even in the absence of bowel or abdominal surgery. Add to this the postoperative ileus induced by handling the GI tract and any electrolyte disturbance as a consequence of surgery, and it is not surprising to discover that nearly everyone feels constipated at some stage after surgery.

For the majority of patients, constipation resolves spontaneously as bowel function returns after surgery. It may be necessary to consider an oral laxative (such as lactulose 20 ml b.d. orally) or, in cases where the patient has faecal impaction, a phosphate enema in order to improve bowel function.

Occasionally a patient with faecal impaction will have overflow diarrhoea and it is important to undertake a rectal examination to ascertain that this is the case. Without the knowledge that the patient is in fact impacted, there may be a temptation to prescribe antidiarrhoeal agents (such as codeine phosphate) when, in fact, the patient needs a gentle enema to start them passing bowel motion normally or, occasionally, a digital emptying of the rectum.

VOMITING

Think

Vomiting is a frequent complaint in the postoperative period. Common causes are certain types of *anaesthetic*, other *drugs* such as opiate analgesia, *infection* and, less commonly but perhaps more seriously, *impaired GI transit* due to abdominal surgery.

As you walk over to the ward, think what operation the patient has and how this might have affected the GI tract. If it is more than 24 h since the patient's anaesthetic, it is unlikely that the anaesthetic will be responsible for their nausea and vomiting.

On the ward

1. Examine the patient carefully, noting any other symptoms associated with their vomiting (pain, nausea, diarrhoea).
2. Examine the patient's abdomen for signs of intestinal obstruction or gastric outlet obstruction.
3. Look at the patient's temperature chart and medication card.

Investigations

- Check that suitable intravenous access is available and take blood for FBC and U & E.
- Order an erect and supine abdominal film.

Management

1. Administer intravenous fluid.
2. Pass a nasogastric tube to empty the stomach contents (see page 173). This is particularly important as postoperative patients are at risk of aspiration of stomach contents. Whilst unpleasant for the patient at the time of passage, the risks of aspiration pneumonia far outweigh any minor unpleasantness in the passage of a nasogastric tube.
3. Administer metoclopramide 10 mg i.v./i.m. t.d.s. or prochlorperazine 12.5 mg/i.m. q.d.s. as an antiemetic, which may further relieve the patient's symptoms.

PYREXIA

Think

A raised temperature (>37°C) frequently occurs in the postoperative patient. It often occurs without associated symptoms and is not a reflection of serious underlying pathology.

- Pyrexia within 24 h of non-infected surgery is virtually never due to infection acquired during surgery. It is most frequently related to the anaesthetic and often due to basal atelectasis after ventilation.
- Pyrexia on days 1–2 is often non-infectious: tissue breakdown, a haematoma, collapse of a lung segment or lobe, or a complication of blood transfusion.
- Pyrexia on days 3–5 is often due to sepsis: wound infection, pelvic or subphrenic abscess, pneumonia.
- Pyrexia on days 5–7 can be due to a leakage or fistula from a failed bowel anastomosis, or from a DVT in the lower limb or pelvic veins.
- Even if you are unable to locate the exact cause of pyrexia during the 'small hours', you can institute simple investigations and treatment.
- Rigors, whilst distressing for the patient and disconcerting for the ward staff, are not a particularly important clinical finding. The haemodynamic status of the patient and signs of septicaemia or localized sepsis are much more reliable indicators upon which to make a clinical assessment and plan management.
- In the surgical patient with sepsis as the cause of a pyrexia, the most common sites for infection are in the chest, urinary tract and abdomen/wound.

On the ward

1. Clarify exactly what operation the patient has had. Establish any operative risks for sepsis.
2. Check for any localizing symptoms (cough/dysuria/calf pain).
3. Examine the patient carefully for localizing signs.
4. Take blood for FBC and blood cultures *before* administering any antibiotics.

> **Remember**
>
> A blood culture taken from a single venepuncture site has only a 60% chance of detecting an organism in the face of bacteraemia. The chance of detecting an organism increases to 75% with two venepunctures and 90% with three.

5. Collect urine and sputum samples for culture.
6. Order a CXR.
7. Institute treatment with appropriate first-line antibiotics once all samples have been collected (see page 210). If chest sepsis is suspected, ampicillin 500 mg q.d.s. may be used; if urinary tract, trimethoprim 200 mg b.d.; and if intra-abdominal, cefuroxime 750 mg t.d.s. with metronidazole 400 mg t.d.s.
8. Chase the results of your cultures and if necessary change your antibiotic therapy in line with the Microbiologist's recommendation.

Longer-term management

In most patients, the above simple approach will solve the problems of pyrexia and sepsis after surgery. In some, however, the cause of sepsis may prove more obscure. Consider:

- Occult septic focus:
  - Abdomen (USS/CT)
  - Heart (repeat blood cultures/ECG)
- Occult infection:
  - Viral illness (viral titres)
  - TB (Mantoux)
- Other disease:
  - Connective tissue disorder (autoantibodies)
- Undiagnosed malignancy, e.g.:
  - Lymphoma
  - Hypernephroma
  - Chronic leukaemia.

PAIN

Think

A patient may have perfectly appropriate postoperative pain which is unbearable because of inadequate analgesia. However, excess pain in the postoperative period may herald postoperative complications which require your intervention.

- Pain may be due to a complication of surgery, such as haemorrhage, perforation of a viscus or arterial embolus/thrombus.
- Common postoperative complications, such as DVT and PE, will also cause pain.
- Abdominal pathology, such as pancreatitis and acute cholecystitis, often occurs after the stress of a major operation and may be particularly difficult to diagnose after abdominal surgery. They should always be borne in mind in a patient who appears more unwell than they should be after an abdominal operation.

On the ward

1. Assess the patient.

> **Remember**
>
> It is often difficult to assess the degree of pain because of patients' differing reactions. Do not be made to panic by the patient who is screaming and thrashing around, but carefully assess their complaint and examine them.

2. Check pulse, blood pressure and temperature.
3. Examine with particular care the area where the patient complains of pain.
4. Investigate as appropriate on the basis of your history and examination.

Investigations

Suspected intra-abdominal pathology

1. Make sure that the patient has good intravenous access.
2. Take blood for FBC, U & E, amylase and cross-match.
3. Order an erect CXR and plain abdominal film.
4. If you are worried that the patient has peritonitis, contact your next on-call to discuss the case.

Peripheral limb ischaemia

1. Having compared your clinical examination with previous postoperative findings, check for peripheral pulses using a Doppler probe.
2. Take blood for FBC, U & E and cross-match.
3. If there has been a deterioration in peripheral circulation, contact your next on-call for advice.

Chest pain (see page 48)

Uncontrolled postoperative pain

1. Check analgesic dosages over the previous 24 h and if the patient is short of analgesia, prescribe appropriately.
2. Double check that you are not missing some other serious pathology as the cause of the patient's pain before ascribing their symptoms to appropriate postoperative discomfort.

> **Remember**
>
> In the case of *unusual aches and pains*, patients may often have joint and back pains related to their stay on the operating table. It is also important to remember that just because a patient is in the post-operative period, it does not preclude them from suffering from a common headache and other such painful complaints.

PAIN RELIEF

Pain is a unique sensation in that, despite its physiological nature, it is primarily a subjective experience which is hard to measure, or even define. As a House Surgeon nearly all your patients will at some point in their hospital stay experience pain either as a consequence of their disease or as a result of their treatment.

You are going to encounter two types of pain:

- Acute pain, due to:
  - trauma
  - surgery
  - inflammatory illness (e.g. pancreatitis)

- Chronic pain, due to:
  - Benign incurable disease (e.g. lumbar disc herniation)
  - Cancer.

Acute pain usually improves over a fairly short time and is relatively easy to treat. Chronic pain, which will either stay the same or get worse, is often very difficult to treat successfully.

Pharmacology

Pain may be managed by a range of drugs (see page 212). There are a huge number of preparations of differing classes of analgesic drugs, which are marketed either as single agents or in combination with other agents.

Administration of drugs

For an analgesic to be effective it must reach the site of action, and this is usually done by getting it first into the plasma.

Oral administration   When a drug is taken by mouth it passes via the stomach into the small intestine and, after absorption, to the liver along the portal vein. The liver is such an efficient metabolic organ that a significant proportion of the drug is usually removed from the plasma and metabolized before it arrives anywhere near the pain pathway ('first pass effect'). This will obviously influence the analgesic effect of a drug given by mouth.

Parenteral administration   This includes intramuscular and intravenous administration. Muscle is a very vascular tissue and a drug injected into it will be absorbed fairly rapidly into the plasma. Because the liver is 'bypassed', plasma concentration will be higher than that achieved by taking the same dose by mouth. Giving drugs directly into the plasma by the intravenous route ensures high plasma levels rapidly.

In an individual patient there will be plasma levels of the drug below which analgesia is not achieved and above which overdosage may occur. For adequate and trouble-free pain relief it is clearly important to maintain the plasma concentration within these limits.

Following a dose of the analgesic drug, the plasma level will rise into this 'therapeutic range' and pain relief will occur. After reaching a peak, the concentration will start to fall and, for the patient to remain comfortable, it is important to give a further dose of the drug before the plasma level falls too low. The timing of intermittent drug administration is determined by the half-life of the drug.

5

Record keeping

Written consent is required for many procedures in hospital. Consent should be obtained by the person performing that procedure; however, as the House Surgeon you will find that it is often your responsibility.

Current trends are towards obtaining consent for more and more minor procedures. Local rules vary but in general it is almost impossible to obtain consent for too trivial a thing. Certainly formal consent must be obtained for all procedures involving anaesthetic or sedation and all procedures which carry a material risk (see below).

Consent means *informed* consent, the patient must *understand*:

- What exactly is going to be done
- Why it is being done
- Any possible alternatives
- The benefits
- Any *material* risks.
  - General: risk of anaesthesia; risks of any operation, DVT, bleeding, infection etc.
  - Specific: recurrent laryngeal nerve palsy after thyroid resection; colostomy in any colonic surgery; conversion to an open operation in any laparascopic procedure; bile duct injury in biliary operations.

If you cannot answer all the questions above you must *not* consent the patient. Don't be afraid to ask either nursing staff or a senior colleague. If you still don't feel able to answer the patient's questions then ask the person doing the procedure to consent the patient; it's their responsibility.

Material risk

Material risks are defined as those to which a reasonable person in the patient's position would be likely to attach significance. Legally a doctor may be deemed negligent if he or she fails to mention a risk which a reasonably competent practitioner in a similar position would have mentioned (the Bolam test). It is good practice to make a short, signed entry in the notes detailing the information you have given to the patient.

> **Remember**
>
> Don't be afraid to ask a senior about the procedure before going to obtain consent, it is your legal responsibility

Consent for testing organ donors for HIV infection

Specific consent should be obtained before a living donor is tested for evidence of HIV infection.

In the case of cadaveric donations, careful enquiries of relatives should be made in a sensitive manner to exclude as far as possible donors at high risk of HIV infection, around the time that consent for organ donation is requested. It should be explained to relatives that assessing the suitability of organs for transplantation will involve testing for certain infections, including HIV.

Relatives who do not wish to be informed of test results If a clinician is satisfied that a positive test has no implications for the health of others, relatives can be assured beforehand that, if they prefer it, the results of tests will not be reported to them.

Donors found to be infected with HIV If a living donor is found to be infected then their organs should not be used and they should be managed as any other patient and appropriate counselling given.

When a cadaveric donor shows evidence of infection with HIV, the implications for the health of sexual partners and, in some cases, children of the deceased will also need to be considered. The question of what information should be given and to whom should be considered on an individual basis by the clinician responsible.

DEATH OF PATIENTS

The death of a patient in hospital triggers a whole sequence of events, many of which are performed by nursing and clerical staff. As the House Surgeon it is your responsibility to complete the following.

Certifying death
You will be required to certify the death of the patient on the ward before the nurses can arrange for the body to be removed and you will be expected to do this at any time of day or night. There's nothing you can do about this, so it makes life a lot easier if you just get on with it.

All you have to do is confirm that the patient is dead! (check respiration, pupil reaction to light and a major pulse) and write in the notes that you have done this, along with the date, time, your bleep number and signature.

Death certification
An altogether different and more complex task than the above. This is the official documentation of the patient's cause of death that must be delivered, usually by the next of kin, to the Registrar of Births and Deaths within 5 days of the death (8 days in Scotland).

Only a doctor who has seen the patient within the 14 days prior to their death can legally fill in the certificate. In order that funeral arrangements are not delayed you should ensure that you fill in the certificate on the morning of the next working day after the death.

The form itself is not the easiest thing to complete. It consists of basic patient details followed by a section about the cause of death (the tricky bit!); this is split into four parts:

- Section 1a is the condition that led directly to the patient's death, e.g. renal failure.
- Section 1b and 1c are conditions that directly led to the condition in 1a, e.g. carcinoma of the bladder.
- Section 2 is for other conditions which, whilst not directly related to the condition in 1a, may have contributed to the patient's demise, e.g. ischaemic heart disease.

The conditions in section 1 should follow in sequence, 1c leading to 1b which leads to 1a which killed the patient. You do not have to fill in all the sections; however, 'organ failures' in section 1a is not acceptable unless qualified by an underlying cause in sections 1b or 1c.

If you are uncertain of what to put, do not be afraid to ask a senior either from your firm or of the hospital's pathology department. If you don't agree with what they tell you then do *not* sign the form; ask them to do it.

Cases which must be referred to the coroner

- Cause of death unknown (this will include most deaths within 24 h of admission)
- Death from criminal, suspicious or unnatural causes (this no longer includes chronic alcoholism)
- Where the patient has not seen a doctor in the preceding 14 days
- Death caused by medical treatment (including those within 24 h of anaesthesia)
- Where the patient has suffered a recent accident or injury, whether or not the immediate cause of death was natural
- Where there is a claim for negligence against hospital staff
- When death occurred as a result of the deceased's employment, e.g. asbestos-related deaths
- Where the deceased was in receipt of a disability or war pension
- Death in custody or whilst detained under the Mental Health Act.

If in doubt, discuss the case with the Coroner's Office.

There are occasions when you cannot fill out a death certificate (see below) and in these circumstances you must contact the local Coroner's Office who will usually deal with all arrangements from then on. If you are uncertain about whether to refer to the Coroner you should call the office where the staff are usually very helpful.

Informing the GP

As soon as possible after a patient's death (usually when you go to fill in the death certificate) you should contact the patient's GP and inform them of the patient's death and any problems associated with it. Families often visit their GP in the days after the death of a relative and the GP will not thank you if he or she has to receive them unprepared.

Cremation forms

The filling in of cremation forms is designed to avoid the cremation of patients for whom the cause of death is uncertain. Coroner's cases cannot be cremated until the Coroner gives his or her permission. There are two parts to the form.

Part one

This is the part that you fill in. The form consists of mainly basic details about the patient and their death. Before going to fill out the form you need to know what was recorded on the death certificate (the cause of death must be the same) and also to have access to the notes for the patient's address and whether they had any operations in the year before their death. It is a legal requirement that you see the patient after death (for the purpose of the form you carry out a 'routine external' examination) and this allows you to confirm that they do not have a pacemaker or radioactive implant, neither of which respond well to being burnt!

Part two

The second part of the form must be completed by a doctor from a different firm who is fully registered and has been qualified for more than 5 years. This is usually one of the hospital pathologists although it is strictly speaking at your invitation. Whoever it is will contact you to confirm the details and if necessary discuss anything they are not happy about.

Both parts of the form carry a fee (currently £38 each). You must keep a record of how many forms you fill in as it is one of the areas the taxman will find particularly easy to cross-check to see whether you have undeclared earnings.

Brain death

Although you are not required to make a diagnosis of brain death, since this must be done by two doctors of Consultant or one of Consultant and one of Senior Registrar status, it is as well to be aware of the criteria.

Preconditions

- Potentially reversible causes for the patient's condition must have been adequately excluded:
  - Drugs: neuromuscular blocking agents, etc.
  - Hypothermia
  - Metabolic or endocrine disturbances.
- Tests for absence of brain stem function must be negative:
  - Eyes: pupillary reaction, corneal reflex, eye movement on caloric testing
  - Motor response: cranial nerve distribution in response to stimulation of face, movements of limbs or trunk, gag reflex, cough reflex.
- Recommendations for apnoea must have been followed-up and the identification of respiratory movements must be made.

The date and time of each testing should be recorded.

Organ donation

Where there is a possibility that a patient has undergone brain death and may be a suitable organ donor, all that is required is that the Consultant's permission is obtained and the local transplant coordinator should be able to do the rest, including, where appropriate, obtaining the permission of the relatives, although you can do this if you feel able.

> **Remember**
>
> Never lose a possible donor because you are afraid to ask.

AUDIT

In many hospitals, active participation in the audit of surgical practice is written into your job description. The House Surgeon's role is usually to collect the basic raw data in the form of audit cards, but may also involve the active physical role of placing these data onto a computer database. In addition, you should also participate in weekly audit meetings, which review your firm's discharges over the last 7 days. The data from these meetings will form the monthly group audit where the work of the firm is peer reviewed.

Such monthly meetings are now essential and must be attended. From January 1990, representatives of the Royal College of Surgeons have inspected both hospital records and audit meeting minutes to ensure that optimum standards of surgical care are being provided for patients. Failure in either of these departments can result in loss of recognition for registration and training purposes.

The hospital records (with reference to the specific guidance of the Royal College of Surgeons of England)
Every patient must have a unique and *personal record* which should contain:

- Patient's name and medical record number on every page and result entry.
- Patient's sex, date of birth, address with postcode and telephone number.
- Person to notify in an emergency.
- Name, address and telephone number of patient's GP.

The *clinical records* of each admission should contain:

- Full history, including details of previous illnesses (including the social and environmental context of these illnesses if relevant) and details of allergies and current medication.
- Details of the physical examination on initial admission.
- Continuing differential diagnosis and medical care plan.
- Each and every entry must be signed and dated in an identifiable way by the appropriate doctor.
- Nursing records and care plan.

When patients *undergo surgery*, the records should include:

- Signed evidence that informed consent has been obtained by a physician, including evidence that the correct procedure has been followed in the case of a minor (under 16 years of age).
- The *medical care plan* should include the site and side of any procedure, written in full and not abbreviated.
- The *operation record* must include:
  - Name of the Operating Surgeon and Anaesthetists, and Consultant responsible
  - Diagnosis and procedure performed
  - Operative findings
  - Details of tissues removed, altered, added
  - Details and serial numbers of prostheses added
  - Description of any difficulties or complications encountered, including how they were overcome
  - Immediate postoperative instruction
  - Surgeon's signature.
- The *anaesthetic record* should include:
  - Anaesthetist's name, and name of Consultant Anaesthetist responsible
  - Anaesthetic preoperative assessment
  - Name, dosage and route of administration of drugs given to induce, maintain and recover from anaesthesia
  - Monitoring data
  - Intravenous fluid therapy
  - Postanaesthetic instruction
  - Anaesthetist's signature.

When a patient is *admitted to ICU*, the record should state:

- Why the patient was admitted to ICU.
- An accurate record of the monitoring of the patient's physiological state while in ICU.
- Records of all therapeutic manoeuvres performed.
- When discharged from ICU, a full description of the patient's clinical status and reasons for the transfer.

Upon *discharge* from hospital:

- All patients must take home with them a brief summary note containing:
  - Name of Consultant in charge
  - Final diagnosis
  - Current medication at discharge
  - Arrangements for local management.
- This should be followed within 14 days by a discharge summary which includes:
  - A précis of the clinical notes
  - Full diagnosis
  - Arrangements for follow-up.

  This summary should be sent to the GP and, if relevant, the referring physician and a copy retained for the notes.

- The first sheet must be completed at the time of discharge, or as soon as the relevant information is available. It should include details of all diagnoses and procedures.

  Your Consultant is responsible for entering a diagnosis and ensuring that the coding process is correct.

When a patient *dies:*

- Similar documentation as for discharge should be completed and sent to the GP.
- Details of the death certificate entry and cremation form entry should be written into the patient's notes.

Postmortem report

- If performed, a provisional diagnosis should be completed in the medical record within 72 h, the final diagnosis and detailed postmortem findings should be completed in the medical notes within 1 month of death.

Collecting the data

Setting up and performing effective clinical audit requires time, effort and financial support. All members of the clinical team and the unit medical secretary must be involved, authoritive and determined if the audit is to work. To be worthwhile, the unit should meet weekly under the chairmanship of the Consultant who will instill the purpose and enthusiasm necessary for good audit.

There is no 'correct' means of collecting clinical data for

audit; the techniques employed must be tailored to the way the clinical office works and discharge information collected and processed. The best way to undertake this is to enter the relevant data onto a specific audit card at the relevant time points during the patient's admission. Ideally the cards should be kept by you separate from the notes and the best place is your white coat pocket. The reason for keeping these cards separate is because invariably when patients die or are transferred to other wards, or remain 'outliers' on other wards for the duration of their admission, the clinical notes never return directly to the clinical office. These cards then form the agenda of the weekly firm audit.

During the weekly meeting, the first priority is to check the accuracy of the data presented. The second priority is to ensure that adequate follow-up has been planned for each patient and, thirdly, this meeting serves as a useful teaching forum. From the data generated and validated by these meetings discharge summaries can be created, often with the aid of complete patient management computer systems, such as 'Micromed'. Entry of these data to the computer is either the responsibility of the clinical secretary or the registrar but may in turn be passed to you. The advantages of medical staff performing this task are: to reduce inaccuracies in data entry, give experience in computer use, and provide instant access to information about patients with full reports of personal operative/clinical experience. Special care is necessary, particularly when entering numerical data such as hospital numbers. All new members of the team should be fully tutored in all aspects of clinical data handling relevant to audit.

Performing the audit

Audit is the systematic appraisal of the implementation and outcome of any process in the context of prescribed targets and standards. Clinical audit should include the access of patients to medical care (appointments, investigations, admissions, waiting times); the process and the outcome of that medical care; and finally the administrative and financial constraints relevant to clinical practice. The result of this process should encourage changes and improvements in clinical practice; provide peer support for the clinician; serve as an educational medium for both seniors and juniors; and ultimately raise the overall quality of clinical care provided in a given department.

Ultimately your Consultant is responsible for initiating and maintaining clinical audit and the week-to-week responsibility for maintaining and supervising the audit usually rests with the College Surgical Tutor for your hospital. However, these meetings should include full, frank and truthful discussion of clinical and administrative problems, which are educational and constructive and result in agreement to act or recommended actions to improve clinical results. Audit meetings should *never* be a witch hunt.

With regard to confidentiality the importance of anonymity cannot be overemphasized since any patient or relative (or their lawyer) can demand access to relevant medical notes, but not the audit minutes. Anonymity of all sensitive data must be effected at the earliest opportunity and all audit meetings should be absolutely confidential within the audit group. Hospital administrators only have access to the general conclusions of clinical audit meetings.

Each audit meeting must be minuted to include a list of those attending, the broad topics discussed and the conclusions and recommendations reached. To this end, College inspection of hospitals demands evidence that effective audit meetings have regularly taken place and all surgical staff have regularly attended. They also seek proof of implementation of recommendations arising from these clinical audits.

As a matter of procedure, the Colleges of Surgeons recommends that junior staff are responsible for the accumulation and presentation of data to each meeting, which should be chaired by Consultants in rotation. Essentially each meeting should address access to treatment, specific issues such as appropriation and compilation of clinical investigations and treatment, use of resources and facilities. Finally each meeting should discuss outcome: generally for all patients presenting with the same condition, but specifically in the case of death and major complications. As part of this, the Colleges considers that quality of life after surgery and degree of patient satisfaction with treatment should also be considered. Although evidence of regular audit is necessary for continued recognition of your post of training, it could also provide a basis for successful medico-legal defence by Surgeons and their juniors who are actively participating in such peer review.

THE DATA PROTECTION ACT (1984)

Owing to the Data Protection Act (1984) every doctor is personally liable to pay compensation for damage caused by inadequate security of information (data) held on people: staff or patients.

> **Remember**
>
> The Act imposes a personal liability so you cannot assume that your Health Authority will pay.

The Data Protection Act (1984) was introduced to protect people from the misuse of information and the use of incorrect information held about themselves.

The Act applies to information that has been or could be mechanically processed, e.g. information held on a word processor, computer or computer printout, and lays down eight principles which those responsible for the information must follow:

- Information should be obtained fairly and lawfully.
- Information may be held for one or more specified and lawful purposes.
- Information shall not be used or disclosed in a way that is incompatible with these specified purposes.
- Information shall be adequate, relevant and not excessive.
- Information shall be accurate and kept up to date.
- Information shall not be held longer than necessary.
- An individual shall be entitled to find out whether information is held on him/her and, where appropriate, to have it corrected or erased.
- It is the responsibility of those who collect such data to undertake security measures to ensure that information is secure from access by unauthorized people, alteration, disclosure, accidental loss and destruction.

In addition the Act requires people who are responsible for the data to register with the Data Protection Registrar. This was completed by 1 May 1986 and after that date it has been illegal to use or process information that has not been registered.

Your responsibilities

Although the Act does not apply to non-computerized data, e.g. paper files, all NHS employees are obliged to respect the confidentiality of personal information whether computerized or not.

While all medical staff are careful about maintaining patient confidentiality, some people have particular responsibilities. If any of the eight principles above relate to you, then you must ensure that you work within these guidelines.

If you hold information on *identifiable* individuals on equipment in your own department or elsewhere, e.g. at home, you must ensure that the information and the use to which it is being put has been registered.

If you operate automatic processing equipment you must ensure that the information it contains is safe and is not accessible in any way by unauthorized people. This means that passwords must be changed regularly, VDU screens checked to ensure that they cannot be seen by passers-by and all demonstrations or training done on 'dummy' data. This is particularly applicable to patient waiting list and audit management systems, such as Micromed.

NOTIFIABLE DISEASES

As of 1 October 1988

UNDER THE PUBLIC HEALTH (CONTROL OF DISEASE) ACT (1984)

Cholera
Plague
Relapsing fever
Smallpox
Typhus

UNDER THE PUBLIC HEALTH (INFECTIOUS DISEASES) REGULATIONS (1988)

Acute encephalitis
Acute poliomyelitis
Anthrax
Diphtheria
Dysentery (amoebic or bacillary)
Leprosy
Leptospirosis
Malaria
Measles
Meningitis
Meningococcal septicaemia (without meningitis)
Mumps
Ophthalmia neonatorum
Paratyphoid fever
Rabies
Rubella
Scarlet fever
Tetanus
Tuberculosis
Typhoid fever
Viral haemorrhagic fever
Viral hepatitis
Whooping cough
Yellow fever

Acquired immune deficiency syndrome

AIDS is *not* a statutorily notifiable disease. Instead, doctors are urged to participate in a voluntary confidential reporting scheme. AIDS cases should be reported on a special AIDS clinical report form *in strict medical confidence* to the Director, PHLS Communicable Disease Surveillance Centre, 61 Colindale Avenue, London NW9 5EQ. Advice about the reporting of cases may be obtained from CDSC (0181–200-6868), or locally from physicians in genitourinary medicine and infectious diseases physicians.

MEDICAL EVIDENCE FOR SOCIAL SECURITY AND STATUTORY SICK PAY

A statement from a medical practitioner is required by the Department of Social Security for claims of incapacity and maternity benefit, and may also be required by employers for statutory sick pay purposes. Any medical question concerning these statements can be raised with your Divisional Medical Officer (Regional Medical Officer in Scotland).

The points you must be aware of are:

- A statement of advice on refraining from work (Form Med. 3) or certificate of expected confinement (Form Mat.B1). This must never be issued without seeing the patient, and never issued more than 1 day after examining the patient. On each and every occasion you must satisfy yourself as to the necessity of the patient staying off work.
- Duplicate statements on the prescribed form can only be issued if the original is lost and then must be clearly marked 'Duplicate'.
- Do *not* sign your statement until the rest of your part of the form is completed. Always sign the certificate in ink.
- The diagnosis of the disorder disabling the patient from work should be entered fully and accurately. This information is also used to compile statistics about disease and disability.
- If the patient is expected to return to work in the next 14 days, then you should issue a 'closed' statement indicating the earliest day during the next fortnight that the patient can return to work. The patient will then not need to consult a physician further before returning to work. A 'closed' statement is made on Form Med.3 by completing Part (b) after 'until', indicating the earliest day within the next 14 days on which you consider the patient fit to return to work.
- Doctors are not required to issue statements for patients of incapacity for work lasting 7 days or less or the first 7 days of longer periods. During this time the patient 'self-certificates'.
- During the first 6 months of absence from work, statements covering formal periods of not > 6 months may be issued. This will not usually involve you. Such matters will usually rest between the patient and their GP. However, it may arise for patients spending protracted periods in hospital, such as young men with major orthopaedic injuries.
- Once a patient has been continuously unfit for > 6 months and recovery in the forseeable future is not expected, the words 'until further notice' can be entered on the statement, as long as such an entry would have no harmful effects on the employment prospects of the patient.

- All remarks entered are at your discretion. You may wish to record that you have or have no doubt about earlier illnesses when you examine a patient some time after the onset of a current illness. This applies equally whether or not you are currently advising the patient to refrain from work.

Essentially you must do the following:

- Every statement is completed in ink with the following particulars:
  - Patient's name
  - Date of examination on which the statement is based
  - Diagnosis of the disorder disabling the patient from work
  - Date on which the statement is given
  - Doctor's signature
  - Name and address of the doctor.
- In the case of an initial examination by a physician in respect of a disorder stated by the patient to have caused incapacity for work, but where there are no clinical signs of that disorder and in your opinion the patient need not refrain from work, then instead of specifying a diagnosis, 'unspecified' can be entered.
- When completing Form Med. 3, *either* section (a) or section (b) must be deleted.
- When issuing an open statement, enter the period during which the patient should refrain from work after the words 'for' in section (b).
- When issuing a closed statement, enter the date on which the patient is expected to be fit to resume work after the word 'until' in section (b).
- For section (a) do *not* use the phrase 'you need not refrain from work' instead of a closed statement.
- Use of 'further notice' after 'until' in section (b) is to be made only when a patient has already been incapable of work for 6 months.
- Form Med. 3 for social security or statutory sick pay purposes is issued *free of charge*.

Surviving on take

6

Major trauma

123

As part of the general surgical team you will invariably be involved in cases of major trauma, such as after a road traffic accident. It is often difficult to know what to do first when a patient clearly has multiple injuries and it is important as you go to the resuscitation room, or the A & E Department, that you remember the ABCDEs of trauma care and identify life-threatening conditions by adhering to this sequence:

A Airway maintenance with cervical spine protection
B Breathing/ventilation/oxygenation
C Circulation
D Disability: neurological status
E Exposure.

Airway maintenance with cervical spine protection

- While the head is clasped to obtain in-line immobilization of the neck, ask the patient his or her name. A logical response with a normal-volume voice indicates a patent airway and oxygenated brain. A non-verbal response or no response at all means a partial obstruction, a complete obstruction or an unconscious patient.
- Without changing the position of the head, apply a rigid collar, sandbags and tape (you will need an assistant). Clear the airway with suction and insert an oropharyngeal airway if there is any sign of airway compromise. Inspect for foreign bodies and facial, mandibular or laryngeal fractures.
- A definitive airway should be established in all unconscious patients and if there is any doubt about the patient's ability to maintain airway patency. It is a good idea to call the anaesthetist on-call early who may decide to intubate the patient to maintain the airway.
- If you are unable to intubate the acutely obstructed-airway patient yourself and there is no anaesthetist around yet, perform a needle cricothyroidotomy (see page 177).

> **Remember**
>
> In general, in a hospital setting, it is not necessary to intubate the patient yourself unless there is no one else available.

Breathing: oxygenation and ventilation

- All injured patients should receive supplemental oxygen.
- Airway patency alone does not assure adequate ventilation. Expose the patient's chest for inspection, auscultation and percussion.
- A tension pneumothorax, flail chest, massive haemothorax and open pneumothorax are dealt with at this stage.

Circulation

- External haemorrhage is identified and controlled by direct manual pressure.
- A rapid assessment of the grade of shock is necessary (see page 88).
- Insert two large-bore cannulae and send blood for cross-match, FBC, U & E and glucose.
- If the patient is peripherally shut down with poor venous filling, consider a cut-down to the saphenous vein or central venous cannulation via the internal jugular vein or subclavian vein (see page 179).
- An initial fluid bolus of 1–2 litres of warmed Ringers lactate is given to an adult.

In the shocked *child*, you have only two attempts to insert a peripheral line. In children of 6 years of age or younger for whom peripheral access is impossible because of circulatory collapse, an intraosseous puncture and infusion is given until other venous access is obtained.

The initial fluid therapy in a child is 20 ml/kg.

Disability

- A rapid neurological evaluation is performed which establishes the level of consciousness, as well as pupillary size and reaction.
- The consciousness level of a patient is graded by an objective scale such as the Glasgow Coma Scale (GCS) (Table 6.1). The GCS can be conducted in under 1 min and need not unduly delay any other aspect of resuscitation. Having made such an assessment it will be much easier to measure the evolution during the subsequent resuscitation and to communicate with the neurosurgeon.

Exposure

Completely undress the patient but prevent hypothermia. Children have a higher body surface to body mass ratio than adults, leading to increased heat exchange. The use of overhead heat lamps or heaters or thermal blankets is recommended.

After the basic resuscitation of a patient (**A**irway maintenance with cervical spine control, **B**reathing, **C**irculation, **D**isability and **E**xposure), ensure that:

- A urinary and gastric catheter is inserted.
- ABGs are obtained.
- ECG leads are attached.
- An AP CXR, AP pelvic X-ray and lateral cervical spine X-ray are obtained in all polytrauma patients.
- The need to perform a diagnostic peritoneal lavage (DPL) or abdominal USS are considered. The surgeon who will possibly do a subsequent operation should perform the DPL.

Table 6.1
Glasgow Coma Scale

	Variables	Score
Eye opening (E)	Spontaneous	4
	To speech	3
	To pain	2
	None	1
BEST motor response	Obeys commands	6
	Localizes pain	5
	Withdraws (normal flexion)	4
	Abnormal flexion (decorticate)	3
	Extension (decerebrate)	2
	None (flaccid)	1
Verbal response	Oriented	5
	Confused	4
	Inappropriate words	3
	Incomprehensible sounds	2
	None	1

The minimum score is 3/15 and the maximum score is 15/15.
Coma is defined as having a GCS score of 8/15 or less.

- The ABCDE sequence is repeated until you have a stable patient. Now you can proceed to the secondary survey.

In the secondary survey, a complete head to toe examination is done to ascertain whether there are any associated injuries.

HEAD INJURIES

After the basic resuscitation, including **A**irway maintenance with cervical spine immobilization, **B**reathing, **C**irculation, **D**isability and **E**xposure, and performance of the necessary adjuncts (see previous page), a complete head to toe examination is done. This is imperative in all trauma because fractures or visceral injuries are frequently missed during the first assessment. Fifteen per cent of patients with an injury above the clavicle will have a C-spine injury and 5% of head injury patients have an associated spine injury. In the case of a head injury it is doubly important to prevent secondary brain damage: any haemorrhage leading to hypotension and hypoxia will compound any brain damage already present in the patient. Normally this should have been dealt with in the primary survey but even peripheral fractures can cause substantial blood loss.

After the initial resuscitation phase you are now able to classify the severity of the head injury into:

- Mild head injury (GCS 14–15)
- Moderate head injury (GCS 9–13)
- Severe head injury (GCS 3–8).

This descriptive classification is useful for practical purposes.

Mild head injury

- Eighty per cent of patients presenting to the A & E Department are in this category.
- A history of brief loss of consciousness is usually difficult to confirm.
- A CT scan should be obtained in all head injury patients in ideal circumstances, especially if there is a history of loss of consciousness, amnesia or severe headaches.
- Obtain a blood-alcohol level and urine toxicology screen.
- The patient should be admitted for observation in the presence of one or more of the following.
  - Abnormal CT scan or no scanner available
  - Skull fracture, CSF leak
  - Confusion or any other depression of the level of consciousness at examination
  - Neurological signs, significant headache, persistent vomiting
  - Difficulty in assessing the patient (alcohol, epilepsy, children)
  - Significant associated injuries or medical conditions
  - No reliable companion at home, unable to return promptly.
- A well-orientated patient who does not meet one of these criteria for admission can be discharged home with a head injury sheet after discussing the need to return if any problem develops.

Moderate head injury

- Definition: this patient may be confused or somnolent but is still able to obey simple commands (GCS 9–13).
- A CT scan is obtained in all patients.
- Admission for frequent neurological observations.
- About 15% of these patients will deteriorate and go into coma; although they are not routinely intubated, treat them as severe head injuries.

Severe head injury

- The most important aspect is early intubation.
- 100% oxygen until blood gases available.
- Organize DPL (contact surgeon) (see page 191) or USS in all hypotensive comatose patients.

A neurosurgical unit should be consulted:

1. In coma, in depression or objective deterioration in conscious level.
2. In focal neurological signs or fits.
3. In disorientation or other neurological disturbances persisting longer than 12 h.
4. In compound or depressed skull fractures.

Brain dead?

Even if a patient appears to be 'brain dead' with a Glasgow Coma Scale of 3 on admission, do not omit to resuscitate them. This is particularly important as the patient's conscious state may improve drastically with a correction of any hypovolaemia or hypoxia. Furthermore, it may be that the only major injury is a head injury and consideration should be given to potential organ donation in these days of heart, lung, liver and kidney transplantation.

THORACIC TRAUMA

Patients who have sustained an injury to the chest may bleed extremely rapidly into both pleural cavities, which can each hold several litres of blood. It is important to remember this when assessing a patient who appears haemodynamically stable on arrival in the A & E department and collapses within 10–15 min of arrival. Basic resuscitation is as described on page 124 and it is particularly important to get blood cross-matched for patients with thoracic trauma and ensure adequate venous access.

Thoracic trauma may be of two types:

- *Penetrating* (such as a stab wound). Such injuries often cause catastrophic haemorrhage due to laceration to major pulmonary vessels, the heart or the great vessels.
- *Blunt* (such as a deceleration injury against a car steering wheel). Such injuries often cause multiple rib fractures and in addition may lead to the avulsion of one of the major vessels. In addition, trauma to the sternum can lead to MI and arrhythmias due to the direct blow to the heart.

Management

Always think of a pneumothorax as a potential complication of thoracic trauma.

1. Do not hesitate to place a chest drain (see page 203) if there are signs of a pneumothorax.
2. Order a portable CXR as a priority. This may show:
   - *Mediastinal widening*: this is indicative of trauma to either the heart or great vessels and such a finding on X-ray

should be followed by consultation with your next on-call and referral to a Thoracic Surgeon

– *Fluid in the pleural cavity* (usually blood): requires a chest drain (see page 203). Patients with a haemothorax require referral to a Thoracic Surgeon

> **Remember**
>
> The initial rush of blood on placing a chest drain does not reflect the rate of haemorrhage. However, once the haemothorax has been drained, subsequent haemorrhage should be measured to gain some assessment of the rate of bleeding.

– *Broken ribs*: in a young fit person, with between one and three fractured ribs and no chest complications, management may be at home with adequate analgesia supplied by a GP. An exception is the patient with a fracture of the first or second rib, which suggests a high-energy injury with possible associated injuries of the head, neck, lungs, spine and great vessels. If in any doubt about the medical state of the patient or their age, or in the presence of three or more fractures, the patient should be kept in hospital to provide them with adequate analgesia, observe their haemodynamic state and encourage respiration with physiotherapy

– *Surgical emphysema*. This results from an airway or lung injury. It is not the subcutaneous emphysema itself but the underlying lesion that needs to be sorted out.

ABDOMINAL TRAUMA

Trauma to the abdomen may be penetrating (e.g. stab wound) or blunt (e.g. as a result of a road traffic accident). Several important points apply to all abdominal trauma.

- Adequately maintain the patient's airway, breathing and circulating volume and assess their conscious state.
- The most important way of assessing a patient's progress after abdominal trauma is by clinical observation of the pulse and blood pressure and abdominal signs.
- Whilst investigation after an abdominal injury may be useful, USS, DPL and a four-quadrant tap may all yield false-positive and false-negative results. The decision to perform a laparotomy after abdominal trauma should be based solely on your clinical findings.
- All *unstable* penetrating injuries to the abdomen will require a laparotomy. Serial clinical examinations are necessary in *stable* penetrating injuries.

- The initial assessment of a young adult with severe concealed haemorrhage (such as in the case of a ruptured spleen) can be misleading because the blood volume may fall by 50% without any change in blood pressure or CVP. This is due to intense vasospasm and there may be a paradoxical bradycardia, possibly vagally mediated. It is therefore imperative that patients who have had severe trauma to the abdomen but who appear well in the first hour after their accident should not be discharged home, but should be kept for observation, thus avoiding potential disaster.

Management

- A patient whose blood pressure is lower than a systolic of 100 mmHg or whose pulse is > 100/min, or who has signs of peritonitis, may well need a laparotomy. Contact your next on-call to discuss the case.
- In addition to basic resuscitation consider plain CXR and plain abdominal film. In general, plain abdominal X-ray is not particularly helpful after abdominal trauma.
- An emergency USS may be extremely helpful as liver, spleen and kidneys are well visualized by the modality and any rupture or displacement of these organs is often picked up by ultrasound. In addition, any collection of fluid or blood may also be localized by ultrasound.
- DPL is done by the surgical team and should be performed in the following cases:
  - Injury to the lower ribs, pelvis or lumbar spine makes a physical examination equivocal
  - A depressed conscious level
  - Injury to the spinal cord
  - USS or CT scan are not available.

DPL is performed by placing a peritoneal dialysis catheter subumbilically in the midline. If no blood is obtained when aspirating, infuse 1 litre warmed Ringer's lactate or normal saline, and place the empty bag on the floor, which allows the fluid to return from the abdominal cavity to the bag.

Send a sample to the lab for erythrocyte and leukocyte counts. A test is positive with more than 100 000 RBCs/mm^3 or more than 500 WBCs/mm^3 and a laparotomy is indicated.

- A four-quadrant tap involves placing a 20 ml syringe with a green needle through the abdominal wall in each of the four quadrants in an attempt to aspirate blood. It is not often helpful as it requires a very large volume of haemorrhage in order to aspirate free blood by this method.

Because of the limitations of investigations, always consider the patient's clinical state first and foremost and regard any information yielded by subsequent investigation as just one piece of information amongst many.

TRAUMA TO THE LIMBS

Trauma to the upper or lower limbs involves injury to four basic tissues:

- Blood vessels
- Bones
- Soft tissue
- Nerves.

These are listed in order of priority. Thus a vascular injury must assume top priority if the limb is to be saved from irreparable damage, whereas soft-tissue and neural injuries may be managed within the first few days of injury rather than the first few hours and are not discussed here.

ARTERIAL INJURY

1. Resuscitate the patient (see page 88).
2. Examine the patient carefully:
   - Check all peripheral pulses and record these clearly in the notes

---

Remember

Particular fractures, or sites of trauma, are associated with arterial injury:

- *Femoral artery* – penetrating injury in the groin or thigh or fracture of the femur.
- *Popliteal artery* – classically trauma to the knee as in severe fracture dislocation.
- *Subclavian artery* – usually associated with penetrating injuries to the upper chest, but occasionally with severe clavicular fracture or traction injuries to the upper limb.
- *Axillary artery* – usually in association with severe fracture dislocation of the humerus.
- *Brachial artery* – fractured humerus.
- *Radial and ulnar arteries* – severe trauma of the wrist.

Remember also that signs such as an expanding or pulsatile haematoma or an arterial bruit may indicate partial disruption of an artery supplying one of the limbs, even if the distal circulation still appears intact.

– Check for any difference in temperature or colour
  between the limbs
– Note also any obvious deformity.

Management

1. Take blood for FBC, U & E and cross-match.
2. Obtain radiographs of the limb concerned, checking for
   fractures.
3. If the distal circulation is impaired secondary to major
   fractures, maintain simple traction to prevent ischaemic
   damage to the limb.
4. All cases of limb trauma with vascular damage will require
   immediate discussion with your senior colleagues in
   General Surgery and Orthopaedics.
5. Further investigate the patient with angiography, either
   preoperatively or on the table during surgery if required
   prior to arterial repair or reconstruction.

BONY INJURY

Detailed discussion of fractures of the limbs is beyond the
scope of this book; however, certain key points should be
remembered:

- Fracture of a major long bone, such as femur, can readily
  cause the loss of 2 units of blood into the thigh. Thus a
  patient with several major fractures may require urgent
  transfusion on admission.
- Fracture of long bones may be associated with arterial
  injury (see page 164). Temporary traction may re-establish
  the circulation to the limb and prevent ischaemic damage.
  In a patient with limb fractures, always be aware of the
  possibility of vascular injury.
- If you are the first medical attendant of a patient who has
  suffered major limb trauma, ensure that in addition to
  basic resuscitation there is good venous access, sufficient
  cross-matched blood and, during your investigation of the
  patient, you order an X-ray of all possible sites of bony
  injury.

7

General surgical emergencies

THE ACUTE ABDOMEN

The most common emergency admission on a surgical firm is a patient with abdominal pain. A wide spectrum of patients will be referred under the heading 'acute abdomen'. These may range from patients who have had intermittent grumbling pain for many weeks through to patients who are moribund, secondary to severe intra-abdominal pathology such as a perforated peptic ulcer. Because of the diversity of patients referred to the hospital with abdominal pain, your initial assessment of a patient suffering from abdominal pain is of the utmost importance.

Initial assessment

1. General appearance:
   - Apparently comfortable
   - Writhing in agony
   - Still as a corpse.

   Colicky abdominal pain may cause a patient to writhe uncomfortably during a bout of pain whilst leaving them relatively comfortable in between episodes of pain. In contrast, patients with peritonitis frequently sit very still, often with knees drawn up to their chest and find any movement painful because of the effect it has on their inflamed peritoneum.

2. Note the patient's age, sex and the length of the history of the abdominal pain.
3. Carefully note associated symptoms. Rather than trying to remember a long list of complaints, it is helpful to think of the GI tract from mouth to anus and consider what other symptoms the patient might suffer. For example, pathology in the oesophagus might cause dysphagia, reflux of gastric contents with symptoms of an unpleasant taste in the mouth, retrosternal pain or heartburn and sometimes vomiting. Also note any urological or gynaecological symptoms.
4. Check for a history of concomitant cardiovascular, respiratory or endocrine disease.
5. Note any previous medical history, in particular abdominal surgery, and list carefully any medication that the patient takes regularly.

Examination

1. Start by taking the patient's hand, measuring their pulse rate and blood pressure and place a thermometer in their mouth to take their temperature.
2. Make a note of any stigmata of possible intra-abdominal pathology – finger nail clubbing, palmar erythema, liver flap, spider naevi, Dupuytren's contracture.

Management of the acute abdomen

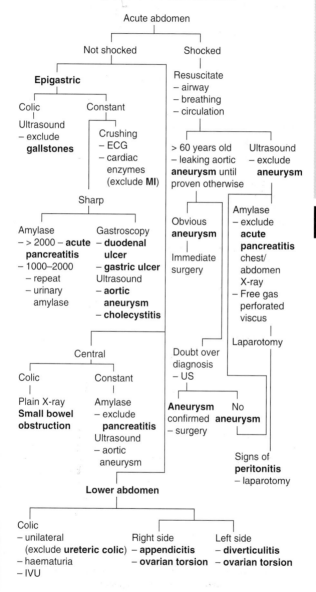

3. Move from the hand to the head and neck area and check conjunctival folds for signs of anaemia and sclerae for signs of jaundice. Feel for a left supraclavicular lymph node (Virchow's node) and move via examination of the chest to the abdomen.

4. Inspect the abdomen:
   – Note previous scars
   – Note any asymmetry in shape and any obvious swelling.

5. Palpate the abdomen:
   – The patient should be relaxed and lying flat with their arms by their side
   – Be gentle and always ask if the abdomen is painful or tender before diving in to a painful examination
   – Gently palpate each quadrant in order starting furthest away from the site of any localized pain
   – Note carefully any areas of tenderness and check for rebound and guarding (signs of peritoneal irritation)
   – Examine systematically the hernial orifices. This is particularly important in obese patients where small inguinal and femoral herniae are easily overlooked. Look specifically for any lump or tenderness in these areas and check for a cough impulse
   – Examine the external genitalia.

6. Feel specifically for the liver, spleen, kidneys and any other masses that you may have detected on your preliminary examination.

7. Percuss the abdomen:
   – This is only necessary if you have made an abnormal finding such as a suprapubic swelling, which if dull to percussion is probably an enlarged bladder.

8. Auscultate the abdomen:
   – Listen to the abdomen for 30–60 s. It is pointless to listen for 2 or 3 s expecting to ascertain the nature of any bowel sounds
   – Normal bowel sounds are detected as an intermittent gentle gurgling sound
   – In a patient with ileus, bowel sounds *may* be more frequent and tinkling in nature as fluid spills aimlessly backwards and forwards in a paralysed bowel
   – In intestinal obstruction, bowel sounds sound very much like a toilet flushing as large volumes of fluid spill from one loop to the other
   – There may be a vascular bruit on auscultation of the abdomen, particularly if the patient has aortic or renal vascular disease.

9. Rectal examination:
   – This is essential in all cases of abdominal pain
   – In addition to information about the anus and perianal examination, rectal examination may reveal carcinoma within the rectum, benign tumours of the rectum, localized tenderness in the pelvis, pelvic masses or

prostatic hypertrophy. Without the possibility of rectal examination, all of these potential pathologies would require multiple high-tech investigation and it is true to say, 'If you don't put your finger in it, you will put your foot in it!'

10. Vaginal examination:
   - Always do it with a female nurse present in the investigation room
   - Always remember to change your glove after a rectal examination
   - This is particularly valuable in females with lower abdominal pain
   - In addition to signs of local sepsis and vaginal discharge, it is possible to examine the pelvic organs by bimanual palpation of the uterus and the adnexa. Using this technique, pelvic masses and pelvic tenderness can be identified.

The sites of abdominal pain and likely pathology are summarized in Table 7.1 and Figs 7.1 and 7.2.

Table 7.1
Sites and possible causes of abdominal pain

Whole abdomen
Generalized peritonitis – secondary to perforated viscus
Intestinal obstruction – colicky pain leading to more constant pain, which is indicative of gut ischaemia and imminent perforation

Right upper quadrant
Biliary colic/acute cholecystitis
Cholangitis – usually with jaundice
Acute hepatitis – often with jaundice
Peptic ulcer disease
Right-sided chest infection with pleurisy
Costo-chondritis – Bornholm disease
Muscular – history of trauma or exercise

Left upper quadrant
Peptic ulcer disease
Pancreatitis
Splenic infarct
Angina
Left-sided chest infection with pleurisy
Costo-chondritis – Bornholm's disease
Pulled muscle – history of trauma or exercise

Table 7.1 (contd)
Sites and possible causes of abdominal pain

Right lower quadrant
Appendicitis
Ovarian pathology
Pelvic inflammatory disease
Meckel's diverticulum
Ureteric colic

Left lower quadrant
Sigmoid diverticular disease
Ovarian pathology
Pelvic inflammatory disease
Ureteric colic

Groin and scrotum
Inguinal or femoral hernia
Ureteric colic
Epididymo-orchitis
Torsion of the testis

Abdominal pain radiating to the back or to the loins
Peptic ulcer disease
Pancreatitis
Abdominal aortic aneurysm
Dissecting aneurysm
Ureteric colic

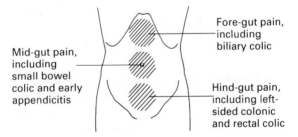

Mid-gut pain,
including
small bowel
colic and early
appendicitis

Fore-gut pain,
including
biliary colic

Hind-gut pain,
including left-
sided colonic
and rectal colic

Fig. 7.1 Sites of visceral abdominal pain.

Initial investigations

- FBC (anaemia, raised white count).
- U & E (electrolyte disturbance secondary to vomiting, diarrhoea or renal insufficiency).

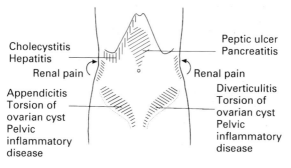

Fig. 7.2 Causes of abdominal tenderness.

- Amylase (pancreatitis).
- Group and save or cross-match (possibility of surgery).
- Urinary dipstick/microscopy (possible urinary infection).
- Erect CXR (lower chest pathology/perforated peptic ulcer).
- Erect and supine abdominal X-ray (intestinal obstruction, ureteric calculi, retroperitoneal abnormality, foreign body).
- ECG (particularly if the patient has cardiac disease or is elderly and surgery is planned).

Initial management

1. Ensure adequate venous access and fluid replacement.
2. Give analgesia (see page 212).
3. Insert a nasogastric tube (see page 173) (if vomiting).
4. Give broad-spectrum antibiotic (see page 210) (if signs of generalized peritonitis and sepsis).
5. Prophylactic subcutaneous heparin (5000 U t.d.s) and stockings for all patients with an acute abdomen.

ACUTE PANCREATITIS

One can be lulled into a false sense of security because most of these patients have a mild self-limiting form of the disease. Some patients will develop cardiovascular, renal and/or respiratory complications and the mortality reaches 20% in the elderly.

Initial assessment

1. General appearance: the pain may be intermittent or steady and vary from mild to severe.
2. History: the majority will have a history of alcohol abuse or gallstones. Less common causes are surgery to the

biliary tract, trauma, virus infections, hyperlipidaemia, hyperparathyroidism and shock with ischaemic injury. A drug history is included (azathioprine, diuretics and other drugs can rarely cause pancreatitis).
3. Note the symptoms: the common presenting symptom is pain which gradually increases in intensity until the patient lies still. Nausea, vomiting and retching are frequent symptoms, often exacerbated by trying to eat. Muscle cramps are late signs of hypocalcaemia.

Examination

1. See page 135: examination of the acute abdomen.
2. The patient becomes hypovolaemic, pale and sweaty.
3. Cullen's sign suggests severe acute pancreatitis; Grey Turner's sign (a bruise in the flank) is caused by acute haemorrhagic pancreatitis.

Initial investigations

1. Pancreatitis is diagnosed on the history and examination. Measurement of the serum amylase can be misleading and should only be used to confirm the clinical diagnosis (if greater than 1200 IU).
2. Free air on an erect AXR confirms a perforated duodenal ulcer. Without free air a differential diagnosis with bowel ischaemia, a perforated duodenal ulcer and even acute cholecystitis is often difficult.
3. USS or CT scan will document gallstones and the status of the pancreas.
4. Baseline blood investigations, serum calcium, ABGs.

Initial management

1. The treatment is supportive once the diagnosis is made: intravenous fluid replacement with colloids, analgesia, nasogastric suctioning, early parenteral feeding.
2. Surgical intervention may be considered if the patient fails to improve.

HAEMATEMESIS AND MELAENA

Upper GI bleeding accounts for between 2 and 5% of all medical and surgical admissions. As a House Surgeon, you will inevitably come across patients who have had either haematemesis (vomiting blood) or melaena (passing altered blood per rectum) (Fig. 7.3). As the first on-call, you must first confirm that the patient has had a GI bleed and then institute basic management before contacting your senior colleagues to discuss further investigation and treatment of the patient.

Initial assessment

1. Has the patient had a significant upper GI bleed? This is

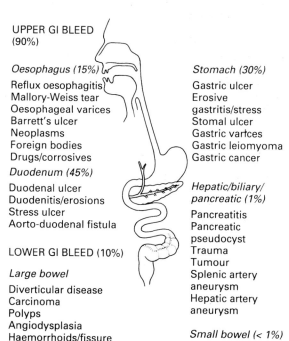

UPPER GI BLEED
(90%)

Oesophagus (15%)

Reflux oesophagitis
Mallory-Weiss tear
Oesophageal varices
Barrett's ulcer
Neoplasms
Foreign bodies
Drugs/corrosives

Duodenum (45%)

Duodenal ulcer
Duodenitis/erosions
Stress ulcer
Aorto-duodenal fistula

LOWER GI BLEED (10%)

Large bowel

Diverticular disease
Carcinoma
Polyps
Angiodysplasia
Haemorrhoids/fissure
Colitis
Ischaemia
Varices
Rectal ulcer

Stomach (30%)

Gastric ulcer
Erosive
gastritis/stress
Stomal ulcer
Gastric varices
Gastric leiomyoma
Gastric cancer

*Hepatic/biliary/
pancreatic (1%)*

Pancreatitis
Pancreatic
pseudocyst
Trauma
Tumour
Splenic artery
aneurysm
Hepatic artery
aneurysm

Small bowel (< 1%)

Meckel's
diverticulum
Tumours
Vascular
malformation
Varices

Fig. 7.3 Causes of GI haemorrhage.

Management of haematemesis

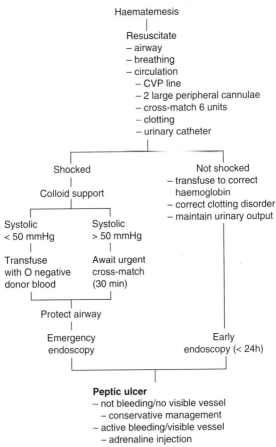

Haematemesis

Resuscitate
– airway
– breathing
– circulation
  – CVP line
  – 2 large peripheral cannulae
  – cross-match 6 units
  – clotting
  – urinary catheter

Shocked

Colloid support

Not shocked
– transfuse to correct haemoglobin
– correct clotting disorder
– maintain urinary output

Systolic < 50 mmHg

Systolic > 50 mmHg

Transfuse with O negative donor blood

Await urgent cross-match (30 min)

Protect airway

Emergency endoscopy

Early endoscopy (< 24h)

Peptic ulcer
– not bleeding/no visible vessel
  – conservative management
– active bleeding/visible vessel
  – adrenaline injection
  – diathermy
Erosions
– manage medically
– continued bleeding: gastrectomy
Varices
– somatostatin infusion
– sclerotherapy
– if fails: balloon tamponade/surgery
Mallory-Weiss tear
– manage conservatively
– torrential bleeding: surgery

defined as > 100 ml, measured or estimated, of fresh or altered blood in vomit or a definite melaena stool.
2. Is the patient hypovolaemic? This is defined as a pulse rate > 100/min or a systolic blood pressure < 100 mmHg or a postural drop in the blood pressure between lying and standing or overt shock.
3. Resuscitation of the patient is the first priority if there are any signs of hypovolaemia. History and examination can be conducted during or after resuscitation of the patient.

Resuscitation

1. Place an intravenous cannula large enough to allow rapid blood transfusion.
2. Take blood for FBC, U & E and cross-match.
3. Start intravenous infusion of normal saline or a plasma expander prior to blood becoming available.
4. Monitor the patient's pulse and blood pressure hourly.
5. CVP monitoring is needed if:
   – The patient is overtly shocked
   – The patient is elderly or unfit and has had a large bleed
   – There is poor peripheral venous access.
6. Aim to maintain the CVP about 5 cm above the sternal angle. A drop of 5 cm or more suggests a re-bleed.
7. Do not allow the insertion of the CVP line to delay essential therapy, such as transfusion, endoscopy or surgery. Do not hesitate to contact a more senior colleague if difficulty is encountered in placing the central venous line (see page 179).

History/examination

1. Document carefully the circumstances of the GI bleed, checking for associated symptoms such as abdominal pain or a change in bowel habit.
2. Make a careful note of any previous medical history which may be of relevance, such as previous peptic ulcer disease and previous GI haemorrhage.
3. Check the drug history for ulcerogenic drugs such as NSAIDs and note whether the patient is taking H_2 antagonists or not.
4. As well as the basic examination involved in your resuscitation (pulse, blood pressure), examine the patient carefully for any signs of intra-abdominal pathology (mass or tenderness) and make sure that a rectal examination is

> **Remember**
>
> Haemoccult testing is useless as a guide to whether a patient has had melaena or not. The most accurate assessment is to look at the stool yourself.

performed, both to assess the macroscopic appearance of the stool and to check for any rectal pathology.

Further management

- Endoscopy. Emergency endoscopy will be required immediately, whatever the time of day in:
  - Patients with overt shock
  - The elderly and unfit, who have had a large bleed
  - Any patient who has had a re-bleed.

  In less urgent cases, endoscopy should be undertaken on the next available list as long as this is within 24 h.

- Indications for blood transfusion:
  - Overt shock
  - Hypovolaemia due to blood loss
  - A haemoglobin < 10 mg/dl.
- Guidelines for surgical intervention in upper GI haemorrhage. Several reports have shown that an acceptably low mortality from all causes of upper GI bleeding can be obtained by instituting a policy of early surgical intervention after the identification of high-risk patients. High-risk patients comprise the following:
  - Patients over the age of 60 years:
    - who require 4 or more units of blood for initial resuscitation
    - who require 8 or more units of blood during the first 48 h of a hospital admission
    - with evidence of active haemorrhage at endoscopy
    - who experience a re-bleed after initial haemorrhage has stopped
  - Patients under the age of 60 years:
    - who require more than 8 units of blood for initial resuscitation
    - who require 12 or more units of blood during the first 48 h of hospital admission
    - with evidence of active haemorrhage at the time of endoscopy
    - who have more than one re-bleed.

> **Remember**
>
> It is important not to be lulled into a false sense of security after experiencing two or three patients admitted with haematemesis and melaena who apparently require very little treatment. Initial resuscitation and cross-match of blood, accompanied by regular observations, will prevent unnecessary mortality from a benign pathology, which is potentially treated either by endoscopic therapy or surgical intervention.

RECTAL BLEEDING

Rectal bleeding may be of four types:

- Fresh blood per rectum is usually the result of pathology between the anal margin and the lower sigmoid colon.
- Blood clots or cherry red blood is indicative of colonic bleeding.
- Melaena or altered blood is usually due to haemorrhage from the GI tract between the oesophagus and the small bowel.
- Occult bleeding is where there are no symptoms suggestive of GI blood loss, but the stool is consistently haemoccult positive and the patient develops recurrent anaemia.

FRESH RED BLOOD

- Haemorrhoids
- Fissure in ano
- Anorectal polyp
- Anorectal carcinoma
- Ulcerative colitis (proctitis)
- Anorectal Crohn's.

Examination

In addition to careful history and examination, the rectum should be examined with a proctoscope and a sigmoidoscope (see page 199) and, if the facility is available, flexible sigmoidoscopy may also be of value.

Investigations

- Take blood for FBC, U & E and cross-match or group and save.
- Order a routine abdominal X-ray.

Management

- Most patients who pass fresh red blood per rectum may be managed conservatively. This involves bed rest with the foot of the bed raised slightly and intravenous fluid replacement as necessary.
- If there is evidence of shock (blood pressure < 100 mmHg, pulse > 100), or persistent haemorrhage on investigation, then more intensive resuscitation may be required and even surgery.

BLOOD CLOTS AND CHERRY RED BLOOD

As mentioned above, this is indicative of colonic bleeding.

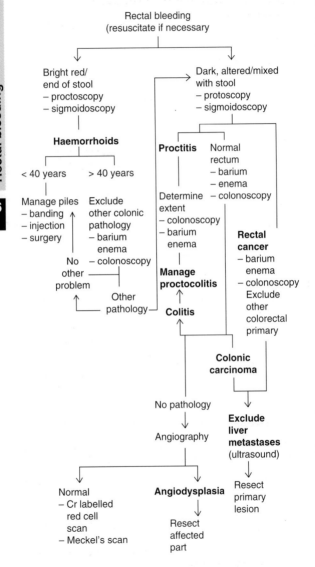

Management of rectal bleeding

Rectal bleeding
(resuscitate if necessary

Bright red/
end of stool
– proctoscopy
– sigmoidoscopy

Haemorrhoids

< 40 years   > 40 years

Manage piles   Exclude
– banding   other colonic
– injection   pathology
– surgery   – barium
                     enema
         No   – colonoscopy
         other
         problem
                    Other
                    pathology

Dark, altered/mixed
with stool
– protoscopy
– sigmoidoscopy

Proctitis   Normal
                     rectum
                     – barium
                     – enema
Determine   – colonoscopy
extent
– colonoscopy
– barium   **Rectal
enema   cancer**
                    – barium
**Manage   enema
proctocolitis**   – colonoscopy
                    Exclude
Colitis   other
                    colorectal
                    primary

**Colonic
carcinoma**

No pathology   **Exclude
                                liver
Angiography   metastases**
                                (ultrasound)

Normal   **Angiodysplasia**   Resect
– Cr labelled   primary
red cell   Resect   lesion
scan   affected
– Meckel's scan   part

History/examination

- In addition to documenting the symptoms leading to the patient's presentation, make a careful note of any alteration in bowel habit, previous episodes of haemorrhage and weight loss.
- In addition to routine examination, perform a rectal examination and sigmoidoscopy (see page 199).

Investigations

As for fresh red blood (see page 146).

Management

- Usually conservative with bed rest and fluid replacement.
- If signs of shock (blood pressure < 100 mmHg, pulse >100), intensive resuscitation with fluid replacement and further investigation by one of the following:
  - Colonoscopy
  - Angiography (blood loss must be > 1 ml/min)
  - Laparotomy with on-table colonoscopy.

MELAENA

See page 142.

OCCULT RECTAL BLEEDING

This is unlikely to present as an emergency but such patients may be encountered as routine admissions as they are investigated. This involves examining the GI tract from oesophagus to anus in order to try and identify the site of blood loss. Ninety per cent of occult blood loss occurs from the upper GI tract, whilst 10% is from the large bowel and lower small bowel (Fig. 7.3).

> **Remember**
>
> As a general rule, lower GI haemorrhage is usually trivial, but once in a blue moon it may be massive and life-threatening.

PERIANAL PROBLEMS

Acute perianal problems commonly present with one or more of the following symptoms:

- Pain

- Lump
- Bleeding.

PERIANAL PAIN

Fissure in ano

Classically presents with pain upon defaecation. It is often difficult to perform a rectal examination upon such patients because of intense pain on introducing your index finger into the anal canal. The fissure is a break in the mucosal lining of the anus, usually posteriorly, and is usually treated surgically, either by lateral sphincterotomy or anal stretch.

Perianal abscess

Commonly presents with perianal pain together with a lump around the anal margin. It may be associated with a fistula in ano (an abnormal tract from the anorectal area to the skin around the anal margin). Treatment is surgical with emergency incision and drainage.

Prolapsed and thrombosed pile

Presents with pain and a tense lump protruding from the anus. Many patients have prolapsing haemorrhoids, but it is only when they become irreducible and their blood supply is cut off, causing them to thrombose, that they present as a surgical emergency. Management may be conservative or surgical. Conservative management includes aperients, bed rest and topical cooling (bag of ice). Surgical treatment is an emergency haemorrhoidectomy.

Ischiorectal abscess

Usually presents with pain and swelling or fullness around the anal margin and is frequently associated with a pyrexia. Management is surgical and involves emergency incision and drainage of the abscess.

Pilonidal abscess

Usually presents with pain and swelling in the natal cleft and around the anal margin. Management is surgical with emergency incision and drainage of the abscess. If it is associated with an obvious pilonidal sinus, attempts should be made to remove this at the time of surgery.

Perianal haematoma

Usually presents with exquisite perianal pain and a small swelling or discoloured area around the anal margin. It may be precipitated by straining stool. Management may be conservative with analgesia and topical cooling or surgical with incision and drainage of the haematoma.

Bartholin's cyst

May be mistaken for perianal pain and swelling. It is in fact an abnormality of the vulva with infection and subsequent abscess formation in one of the glands of the vulva. Management is surgical, involving emergency incision and drainage.

PERIANAL LUMP

A perianal lump on its own rarely leads to emergency admission. In the absence of pain or haemorrhage, most perianal problems will present to the outpatient clinic rather than the emergency room.

Perianal lumps may be caused by:

- Perianal abscess (see page 148).
- Thrombosed or prolapsed pile (see page 148).
- Ischiorectal abscess (see page 148).
- Pilonidal abscess (see page 148).
- Perianal haematoma (see page 148).
- Perianal skin tags – these are not usually the cause of acute symptoms and may be associated with more serious GI pathology such as Crohn's disease or localized disease such as haemorrhoids.
- Perianal warts – usually sexually transmitted and not often the cause of emergency admission.

PERIANAL HAEMORRHAGE

Haemorrhoids

Often lead to spotting of fresh red blood on the toilet paper after defaecation. Haemorrhoids may also be the cause of more significant rectal bleeding. In addition, it is important to remember not to attribute rectal bleeding to haemorrhoids until more serious pathology such as rectal or colonic carcinoma has been excluded. Management of haemorrhage from haemorrhoids is conservative in the first instance. Should haemorrhage prove substantial, see page 148 for management of rectal bleeding.

Fistula in ano

Often presents with perianal irritation, discharge and occasionally slight haemorrhage. Management of a symptomatic fistula in ano is surgical with elective laying open of the fistulous tract, which then allows it to granulate from the bottom up and heal completely.

Pruritis ani

Often presents with irritation, discharge and haemorrhage secondary to overzealous scratching. Management is medical and should not involve any creams or lotions but simply twice daily bathing with water to keep the area clean and dry.

8

Urological emergencies

151

Retention of urine may be acute, chronic or acute on chronic. Patients with chronic retention do not usually present as a surgical emergency unless they go into acute retention.

History

1. Check if there is a previous history of chronic retention, including symptoms of a poor urinary stream, urinary frequency (sometimes leading to nocturia) and intermittent UTI.
2. Ask specifically whether the patient has experienced haematuria.

Examination

1. As well as your general examination, look specifically for signs of an enlarged bladder, which may be difficult to palpate but easier to percuss as a dull area suprapubically.
2. Perform a rectal examination. If the patient is in acute retention defer this until after urinary catheterization has been achieved because the enlarged bladder may make examination of the prostate and surrounding tissues difficult per rectum.

Catheterization

1. Provide the patient with analgesia prior to catheterization.
2. Use a 14 or 16 French urinary catheter and attempt urethral catheterization in the first instance (see page 174).
3. If urethral catheterization fails and the patient has an enlarged percussable bladder, then perform suprapubic catheterization (see page 177).
4. If you have failed to pass a catheter per urethra, and the patient does not have an enlarged bladder, or you are unhappy about suprapubic catheterization, contact your next on-call with a view to either:
   – Introducing a catheter per urethra using a catheter introducer, or
   – Performing an ultrasound scan to confirm a bladder residual volume and to facilitate suprapubic catheterization.

Investigations

- Take urine for microscopy, culture and sensitivity.
- Take blood for haemoglobin, U & E and acid phosphatase (acid phosphatase may be raised in prostatic cancer), PSA.
- CXR – particularly important in elderly patients who may be considered for surgery.

- ECG – similarly important if the patient is to undergo surgery at any stage during their admission.
- USS or intravenous urogram – images the urinary tract from the calyces in the kidney to the bladder and may identify unusual causes of urinary retention, such as carcinoma of the bladder.
- Cystoscopy – may identify a urethral stricture and allow treatment of such a stricture.

Differential diagnosis for acute retention

- *Benign prostatic hypertrophy*
  - Most common cause.
- *Carcinoma of the prostate*
  - May be detected clinically because of a hard knobbly prostate or, on investigation, a raised PSA or acid phosphatase or signs of chest and bony metastases on plain X-rays.
- *Carcinoma of the bladder*
  - May be detected because of a previous history of haematuria, on USS or on finding a filling defect in the bladder on an IVU.
- *Urethral stricture*
  - May be detected if the patient gives a history of previous strictures or urological procedures
  - May be suspected if a urinary catheter appears to get stuck in the penile urethra rather than the prostatic urethra
  - May be detected and treated at cystoscopy.
- *Neurogenic bladder*
  - May be suspected if the patient has intercurrent illness, such as diabetes.
- *Prolapsed intervertebral disc*
  - May be detected if there are neurological signs or a history of backache.

HAEMATURIA

Haematuria presents as an emergency when it is macroscopic, because clearly at this stage it is disturbing to the patient. The majority of cases of haematuria are microscopic and may go unnoticed for many months until they are picked up either because of anaemia, leading to investigation, or because an episode of macroscopic haematuria occurs.

MACROSCOPIC HAEMATURIA

History

Is the haematuria associated with any other symptoms such as dysuria, frequency, loin pain, rigors?

- Haematuria associated with dysuria and frequency may indicate UTI or prostatic infection, either as the cause of haematuria or coexisting with haematuria from another cause such as malignancy.
- Slight haematuria associated with loin pain may indicate a ureteric calculus.
- Haematuria with no other urinary tract symptoms is often due to urinary tract malignancy.

Examination

1. Check for signs of hypovolaemia: pulse and blood pressure.
2. Examine the abdomen paying particular attention to any renal masses or bladder enlargement.
3. Perform a rectal examination to examine the prostate.
4. In women, perform a vaginal examination to palpate the bladder bimanually.

Investigations

- Urine for microscopy, culture and cytology.
- Take blood for FBC and U & E. If the patient is haemodynamically stable, group and save them; if there are any signs of hypovolaemia, cross-match them with a minimum of 2 units of blood.
- Undertake routine plain abdominal film looking for ureteric calculi. Order a routine CXR – this is important if the patient is to undergo surgery and also may show lesions associated with renal pathology, such as cannon ball secondaries from a hypernephroma.

Management

1. Place a ureteric catheter in the emergency admissions area. This is placed for two reasons:

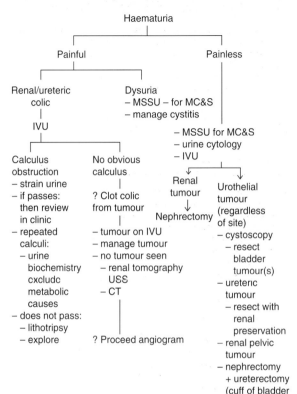

Management of haematuria

Haematuria

Painful

Painless

Renal/ureteric colic

Dysuria
– MSSU – for MC&S
– manage cystitis

IVU

– MSSU for MC&S
– urine cytology
– IVU

Calculus obstruction
– strain urine
– if passes:
    then review
    in clinic
– repeated
    calculi:
    – urine
        biochemistry
        exclude
        metabolic
        causes
– does not pass:
    – lithotripsy
    – explore

No obvious calculus

? Clot colic
from tumour

– tumour on IVU
– manage tumour
– no tumour seen
    – renal tomography
        USS
    – CT

? Proceed angiogram

Renal tumour

Nephrectomy

Urothelial tumour (regardless of site)
– cystoscopy
    – resect
        bladder
        tumour(s)
– ureteric
    tumour
    – resect with
        renal
        preservation
– renal pelvic
    tumour
– nephrectomy
    + ureterectomy
    (cuff of bladder
    included)

– To permit washout of the bladder
– To prevent the patient going into clot retention.
2. Investigate all patients with macroscopic haematuria
   further by means of:
   – USS or intravenous urography
   – Cystoscopy.

The reason for further investigation is to identify causes for haematuria within the renal tract. These may be anything from renal cell carcinoma to transitional cell carcinoma (anywhere from the renal calyces to the bladder). In addition, cystoscopy will eliminate rarer local causes in the urethra, prostatic urethra and bladder.

DYSURIA AND FREQUENCY

Patients do not usually present as emergencies when suffering from urinary frequency, but pain on micturition associated with urinary frequency may cause emergency admission. The most common cause for such symptoms is UTI.

Remember

UTI is much more common in women than men and is more frequent in the very young and the very old.

History/examination

- Infection in the kidney produces pain in the loin frequently associated with rigors.
- Infection in the bladder is usually heralded by suprapubic pain, frequency of micturition and pain on micturition. It is rarely accompanied by septicaemia and rigors.

Investigations
It is difficult to know where to draw the line when investigating such a common condition as UTI:

- All males with evidence of upper UTI should be thoroughly investigated to identify any structural damage or underlying anatomical abnormality which has caused UTI.
- Females who have had two or more previous attacks should also be investigated.
- During a routine admission:
  - Take urine for microscopy and culture
  - Take blood for FBC, U & E and blood cultures (if there are signs of systemic sepsis).

Management

- Having taken urine and blood cultures if indicated, start empirical treatment with trimethoprim 200 mg b.d. orally for lower UTI.
- For upper UTI, start treatment with a broad-spectrum antibiotic such as cefuroxime 750 mg t.d.s. i.v. for the first 24 h of treatment and continued orally thereafter.
- Quantitative microbiological investigation of urine.
- USS or intravenous urography.
- Cystoscopy.

URETERIC COLIC

Stones within the urinary tract most frequently present with pain. They may also present with recurrent UTI or haematuria.

History

- A stone in the *renal pelvis* that impacts in the pelvi-ureteric junction will cause loin pain, often associated with pyrexia.
- A stone in the *ureter* will give rise to colicky loin pain that radiates around to the groin and scrotum. This pain may be associated with dysuria and frequency and haematuria.
- A stone in the *bladder* often presents with pain referred to the tip of the penis. The pain is associated with frequency, dysuria and haematuria.
- *Ureteric calculi* are common and often present after a period of dehydration or prolonged recumbency. In addition, ureteric calculi may be familial, as in the case of cystinuria, or associated with other conditions such as gout. Excessive intake of alkalis or aspirin-related analgesics may also predispose to urinary calculi. It is, however, important to remember that the majority of urinary calculi present in patients with none of these predisposing factors.

Investigations

- Take urine for microscopy and culture and test urine for blood.
- Take blood for FBC, U & E, uric acid and calcium.
- Perform plain abdominal film followed by emergency IVU. The detection rate for ureteric calculi is much higher if the IVU is performed during the acute attack, rather than 48 h later.

Management

- Analgesia
  - The use of an intramuscular NSAID, such as diclofenac 75 mg 12 hourly, is recommended as the best first-line analgesic for patients with ureteric colic.

- Antibiotics
  - If there are signs of lower UTI, oral trimethoprim
    200 mg b.d. should be used
  - If there are signs of upper UTI, cefuroxime 750 mg t.d.s.
    i.v. should be used.
- Most ureteric calculi pass spontaneously. However, in the
  presence of obstruction and infection it may be necessary
  to remove calculi as an emergency. The practice of
  removing a stone by open operation is now very
  uncommon and stones are usually removed by a
  combination of percutaneous and cystoscopic manipulation
  of the ureter. In addition, where centres have a lithotripter,
  extracorporeal shock wave lithotripsy is also effective in
  shattering renal calculi.

THE PAINFUL SCROTUM

Acute pain and swelling of the scrotum and its contents is a
common surgical emergency. Its importance lies in the fact that
one potential cause of such symptoms is torsion of the testis.
Testicular torsion is where the testis rotates on the spermatic
cord, causing the blood flow to the testis to be cut off and
leading to ischaemia and necrosis. Testicular torsion should
be dealt with surgically within 1 h of admission to hospital in
order to prevent necrosis of the testis.

Differential diagnosis

- *Torsion of the testis*
  - May occur at any age, though most often seen around
    puberty
  - Often preceded by severe attacks of pain in the testicles
    coming on suddenly and disappearing just as suddenly
  - Examination of the contralateral testis may reveal that it
    is very freely mobile and lies horizontally rather than
    vertically
  - If this diagnosis is suspected, surgery should be
    performed immediately with a view to fixing both
    testicles to the scrotum to prevent further torsion.
- *Torsion of the hydatids of Morgani*
  - Caused by torsion of one of the remnants of the
    Mullerian duct
  - Often difficult to differentiate from testicular torsion
  - Because of its similarity to testicular torsion it is usually
    dealt with by emergency surgery at which the torted cyst
    is removed.
- *Trauma to the testicle*
  - Remember that one in five testicular tumours present
    after trauma, possibly because the tumour changes the
    size of the testicle making it more prone to injury

- Trauma may lead to a haematocele or a reactive hydrocele which may require drainage
- Trauma may lead to disruption of the testicle itself which may require surgical attention
- USS of the testicle is the best modality of investigation when assessing the organ after trauma. It can confirm any damage to the testicle, the presence of a testicular tumour and the site and size of any fluid collection which may need draining.

- *Epididymo-orchitis*
  - Acute orchitis may occur in association with acute viral infection, such as mumps
  - Acute epididymitis may occur secondary to UTI or prostatitis. Alternatively, it may be due to blood-borne spread after bacteraemia
  - If there are symptoms of UTI and you are certain that the patient has not had a testicular torsion, treatment is with oral antibiotics
  - If there is a reactive hydrocele which makes examining the testis difficult or you are worried about underlying torsion or tumour, undertake a USS or emergency surgery to explore the scrotal contents.

- *Hydrocele and epididymal cyst*
  - These rarely present as emergencies as in the majority of patients they form a swelling without pain
  - A hydrocele is a collection of fluid in the tunica vaginalis around the testis and, as such, it makes examination of the underlying testis impossible
  - An epididymal cyst is found in the epididymis which lies behind the testis. In patients with an epididymal cyst, it should therefore be possible to feel the testis and the cyst in the epididymis behind the testicle
  - Ultrasound examination of the testis is useful both in identifying the underlying testis in a hydrocele and delineating the extent of any cysts in the epididymis.

- *Varicocele ('lover's nut')*
  - A varicocele is a varicose vein of the pampiniform plexus
  - Large bulky painful veins around the spermatic cord should be removed if causing severe symptoms
  - The same symptoms as experienced chronically by the sufferer of a varicocele may be experienced acutely secondary to engorgement of the testicular veins brought on by sexual excitement. Such patients frequently present to the A & E department with acute testicular pain radiating to the right groin. This occurs in the absence of any overt physical signs in the scrotum or right iliac fossa, but is often mistaken for more serious disease, such as appendicitis
  - Management of this condition is a scrotal support and reassurance.

PENILE PROBLEMS

Several penile problems are encountered frequently by the House Surgeon. These are phimosis, paraphimosis and penile inflammation. In addition, the rarer problems of trauma and priapism may often first be encountered by the House Surgeon.

PHIMOSIS

- May present as a problem in emergency surgical admissions for whom a catheter is required and the foreskin cannot be retracted.
- If the need for a catheter is urgent and the placement of a suprapubic catheter is not appropriate, then a dorsal slit under local anaesthetic should be performed, which will allow access to the glans for placement of a urinary catheter.
- Elective circumcision may be required after the patient's other surgical problems have been overcome.

PARAPHIMOSIS

- Paraphimosis is most frequently encountered in patients who have a urinary catheter in place.
- If the foreskin is not pulled back over the glans after placement of a urinary catheter, it may become inflamed and constrict the base of the glans causing acute pain.
- If it proves impossible to return the foreskin over the glans then a dorsal slit should be undertaken as a temporary procedure to relieve the constriction.
- Elective circumcision may be required after the patient's other surgical problems have been overcome.

INFLAMMATION

- Most inflammation associated with urethral discharge in the male is due to sexually transmitted disease and such patients should be referred to the local sexually transmitted disease clinic.
- Severe external inflammation of the glans may be due to rare causes such as balanitis xerotica obliterans or simply allergic dermatitis. Carcinoma of the glans should be suspected if a patient is seen with what appear to be abnormal tissues on the glans.

PRIAPISM

- This is a rare condition caused by impairment of the

venous drainage of the penis leading to failure of an erection to relax.
- Its management is complex and patients should be referred to a senior colleague with urological experience.

TRAUMA

- Minor trauma to the penis may be caused by trouser zips or other such articles of clothing. These rarely cause damage to the underlying structure of the penis or excessive blood loss.
- Such injuries may be managed in the A & E Department and may at worst require excision of a small patch of skin entrapped in the zip under local anaesthetic.
- More major trauma to the penis, such as after a major industrial accident or road traffic accident, may cause quite severe haemorrhage. In such cases, consult a senior colleague immediately to advise on further management of the patient.

9

Arterial emergencies

163

Arterial emergencies arise as a result of vascular occlusion or vascular rupture. In cases of occlusion it is important to establish the timing of events whilst in cases of rupture, emergency surgery is almost always needed.

OCCLUSION

Occlusion of arteries may take place gradually, as in atherosclerosis, or suddenly, as after embolism. Patients usually present as an emergency when there has been sudden vascular occlusion. The management of chronic vascular occlusion is dealt with on page 33; acute occlusion is considered below.

History

- Establish carefully the timing of events.
- Ask about symptoms prior to the acute event, e.g. claudication distance.
- Check for previous surgery, ischaemic heart disease, cerebrovascular disease.
- Ask about smoking habits, other illnesses such as diabetes, and regular medication.

Examination

1. Assess general state
   - Pulse
   - Blood pressure.
2. Document peripheral pulses carefully:
   - Radial
   - Brachial
   - Carotid
   - Aortic
   - Femoral
   - Popliteal
   - Posterior tibial
   - Dorsalis pedis.
3. Check for arterial bruits:
   - Carotid
   - Aortic
   - Renal
   - Femoral.
4. Check for *source of potential emboli*:
   - Atrial fibrillation
   - Cardiac murmurs.
5. Assess *degree and level of ischaemia*:
   - Temperature of limb
   - Sensation
   - Capillary return
   - Venous guttering.

6. Record *Doppler pulse pressures* – after completing a routine clinical examination it is important to establish the presence of pulsatile flow in blood vessels which are not palpable and this is best done using a Doppler probe.

Investigations

- Routine bloods – FBC, U & E, glucose and cross-match.
- Plain AXR and CXR.
- Arteriography may be indicated in situations where there is diagnostic doubt and reconstructive surgery is considered necessary as an emergency. It will delineate any longstanding vascular disease as well as clarifying the level of vascular occlusion. In the presence of history and examination suggestive of simple embolism without previous vascular disease, arteriography is *not* indicated.

Management

- Anticoagulation with heparin (see page 214).
- Peripheral arterial embolism: embolectomy.
- Acute in-situ thrombosis: emergency thrombectomy or intra-arterial streptokinase.
- Acute-on-chronic thrombosis: emergency thrombectomy ± arterial bypass grafting.

RUPTURE

Arterial rupture is most commonly encountered when there is an aneurysm of the abdominal aorta. The first priority when rupture of an abdominal aorta aneurysm is suspected is re-suscitation and immediate surgery. Resuscitation is dealt with on page 88. Once cross-matched blood is available, emergency repair of a leaking aneurysm should be undertaken without delay.

SECTION 3

Surviving in practice

10

Practical procedures in surgery

SITING AN INTRAVENOUS CANNULA AND SIMPLE VENEPUNCTURE

These procedures will be asked of you every day during your house year; the basic outlines are detailed below but success only comes with practice. Don't be put off if you fail initially; after two attempts call for help from a more experienced colleague – they will have done the same in the past!

You will need

- A tourniquet
- An alcohol swab
- A piece of cotton wool/gauze
- In debilitated patients, a piece of tape.

For siting an i.v. cannula

- Cannula 16–22 gauge
- Cannula dressing
- A 2 ml syringe filled with sterile saline solution.

For simple venepuncture

- Appropriately sized syringe – if in doubt take too much!
- Green 20-gauge or blue 18-gauge needle.

Many hospitals use 'Vacutainer' systems, which allow blood to be drawn up directly into the sample bottle. You will probably find a syringe and needle easier in difficult cases.

Preparation

1. Apply the tourniquet on the upper arm, midway between the elbow and the shoulder. Allow up to 5 min for the veins to engorge.
2. Examine for veins by looking and feeling. For simple venepuncture the antecubital fossa is often best; however, this should be avoided when siting a cannula, except in an emergency. Common sites for cannula insertion are the cephalic vein over the distal radius, the dorsal arch on the back of the hand and the proximal branches of the cephalic and median veins in the forearm. The key to success is taking time to choose the correct vein. The best vein is one you can feel, not the one you can see!
3. Clean the selected area with the alcohol swab and allow this to dry.

For siting an i.v. cannula

4. Identify an entry point either 1 cm distal to the join between two tributaries or just to one side of a straight section of the vein.
5. Advance the cannula until you feel a 'give' or see blood flash back at the hub of the needle.

6. Holding the hub of the needle still, advance the cannula over it and into the vein.
7. Release the tourniquet and press on the vein just proximal to the innermost end of the cannula. You can now remove the needle fully and either connect a pre-prepared giving set and infusion or cap of the cannula and flush it with 2 ml of sterile saline via the side port.
8. Finally secure the cannula with a dressing and, if necessary, a bandage (strongly advised in confused patients).
9. Dispose of your sharps carefully.

For simple venepuncture

4. Place the needle on the syringe and insert the needle with the bevel facing upwards at an angle of about 30° into the vein.
5. As you enter the vein you will see a blood flash at the hub of the needle.

> ### Tips and problems

- *Selection of cannula*: for most purposes a pink 20-gauge cannula is adequate. For patients requiring blood transfusion or who are potentially haemodynamically unstable, a green 18-gauge or preferably grey 16-gauge cannula is required. Patients with fragile or fine veins may warrant the use of a blue 22-gauge cannula.
- *Taking blood through a venflon*: this is only possible at the time of insertion and with larger veins but is a useful time saver. Before removing the tourniquet, apply pressure to the vein as described above, remove the needle and insert the syringe into the end port. Release the pressure and carefully aspirate. Gently tapping the vein may aid blood flow.
- *Poor veins*: place the patient's forearm into a bowl of warm water and wait at least 5 min. A sphygmo cuff can be used as a more efficient tourniquet, or if all else fails examine the patient's feet for veins.
- *Thrombophlebitis*: resite the cannula and, if required, prescribe an oral NSAID; topical preparations have no proven benefit.
- *Unable to get blood*: consider a femoral stab, pass the needle vertically downwards immediately medial to the femoral pulse until you aspirate dark venous blood. Apply pressure manually for 2 min.
- *Nervous or young patients (not < 1 year)*: apply Emla cream over a visible vein and under an occlusive dressing, preferably on more than one limb. The vein is constricted after 1 h and dilated after 2 h, so wait 2 h to take blood if possible – the skin will still be numb.

6. Advance the needle a couple of millimetres further and slowly aspirate blood into the syringe. If flow stops, try pulling the needle out slightly whilst aspirating.
7. Once you have enough blood, release the tourniquet.
8. Remove the needle and quickly apply pressure to the site with a piece of cotton wool or gauze. It is preferable for the patient to press on the site for 1–2 min; however, if this is not possible, secure the cotton wool with a piece of tape.
9. Dispose of your sharps carefully and decant the blood into the relevant sample bottles without delay to prevent clotting.

ARTERIAL PUNCTURE (BLOOD GASES)

Indication

- Arterial gas measurements (ABGs).

You will need

- A 21-gauge (green) needle and 2 ml syringe containing 100 U of heparin
- Alcohol swab and a blind syringe hub
- An assistant.

Radial stab

1. Perform the Allen test to confirm the competence of the ulnar artery. Use two fingers to compress the radial artery at the wrist while the patient opens and closes his hand several times. This will cause a transient blanching which should rapidly correct if the ulnar artery is patent. Document the result in the notes.
2. Clean the area with the alcohol swab.
3. Palpate the artery with two fingers.
4. Pass the needle vertically down between your two fingers.
5. When you hit the artery the syringe should fill by itself due to arterial pressure.
6. Remove the needle and ask your assistant or the patient to compress the artery for at least 3 min.
7. Expel any air bubbles from the syringe, remove the needle and cap it off.
8. Transfer the sample on ice directly to the lab; it is often best not to rely on portering staff for this.

Femoral stab

1. Locate the femoral pulse at the mid-inguinal point (midway between the anterior superior iliac spine and the symphysis pubis) (Fig. 10.1).

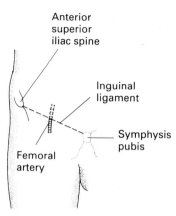

Fig. 10.1 Site of the femoral artery: mid-inguinal point.

2. Place the index and third finger of your non-dominant hand either side of the pulse and press to fix the artery.
3. Pass your needle between these two fingers, vertically downwards through the artery, so transfixing it.
4. Gently withdraw the needle and as it passes back through the lumen of the artery, the arterial pressure will cause bright red arterial blood to fill the syringe.
5. Remove the needle and ask your assistant or the patient to compress the artery for at least 3 min.
6. Expel any air bubbles from the syringe, remove the needle and cap it off.
7. Transfer the sample on ice directly to the lab, it is often best not to rely on portering staff for this.

> **Tips and problems**
>
> *Abnormal clotting*: this does not preclude arterial puncture; your assistant will have to compress the arterial puncture site for longer (upwards of half an hour).
>
> *Totally deranged clotting/DIC*: avoid arterial puncture.

PASSING A NASOGASTRIC TUBE

Indications

- Postoperative gastric decompression
- Persistent paralytic ileus

- Intestinal obstruction
- An adjunct to enteral nutrition.

You will need

- A suitably sized NG tube (size 10–12 French), which has been chilled in the ward refrigerator to stiffen it
- A pair of gloves
- KY lubricating jelly + lignocaine throat spray
- A bladder syringe
- A stethoscope
- Litmus paper
- An assistant.

Procedure

1. Spray throat.
2. Grease the end of the tube with the KY jelly and pass it into the patient's nostril and horizontally along the floor of the nasal cavity.
3. Tip the patient's head slightly forwards and ask them to swallow. The tip of the tube should now enter the pharynx.
4. As you continue to advance the tube it should engage the hypopharynx and, with the swallowing action, enter the oesophagus. Continue to advance the tube until more than 60 cm of tube has been passed.
5. Check the position of the tube by:
   - Aspirating gastric contents, which should be acid when tested with litmus paper
   - Auscultate the stomach while your assistant injects air down the tube; you should hear air bubbling.

> ### Tips and problems
>
> *Patient won't swallow*: try again while at the same time they are swallowing sips of water.
>
> *Meet resistance in the oesophagus*: give up. This tube needs to be passed under radiological control. This may particularly be the case with fine-bore feeding tubes.

URETHRAL CATHETERIZATION

Indications

- Monitoring urinary output, particularly peri- and post-operatively
- Acute urinary retention

- Chronic urinary retention
- Incontinence
- Facilitation of abdominal (particularly pelvic) surgical procedures.

You will need

- A Foley catheter (size 12–16 French), syringe and 10 ml of water already drawn up (check volume of balloon on individual catheters)
- A sterile catheter pack containing drapes
- Antiseptic cleansing solution
- Lignocaine jelly
- A urinary collecting system
- An assistant is helpful but not essential
- A relaxed and reassured patient.

Procedure

1. With the patient supine on the bed, clean the genital area. In a man retract the foreskin and clean around the glans. In a woman, ask her to open her legs, supporting her knees by placing the soles of her feet together. With the fingers of your left hand gently lift and retract the labia to expose the urethral meatus. Place the drapes around the genitals.
2. Gently inject the urethra with the sterile lignocaine jelly and wait 3 min.

> **Tips and problems**

Unable to pass the catheter? Call for help. Do not keep on trying to pass it yourself; there may be strictures or false passages and these require an expert.

Passed the catheter but no urine comes out? The tip may still be smeared with lubricating jelly. Gently inject 5–10 ml of water up the catheter. Urine should then flow back. If nothing happens, either you are in a false passage or the patient is anuric. Do *not* inflate the balloon; call for help.

When *deflating a bladder* which is grossly distended following chronic urinary retention, let the urine out slowly by intermittently clamping the catheter. Release 200–300 ml every 30 or so minutes as rapid decompression may result in haemorrhage from the bladder mucosa. Once the bladder is empty, monitor the urine output hourly, as these patients will get a brisk diuresis over the subsequent 72 h after the back pressure is taken off the kidneys. They can very easily become dehydrated if these urinary losses are not compensated by using crystalloid (see page 224).

(a)

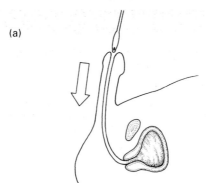

(b)

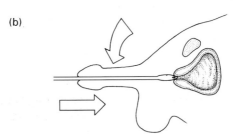

Fig. 10.2 Male urethral catheterization. (a) Initial direction; (b) downward deflection to guide catheter through urethral angle at the junction of the membranous and prostatic urethra.

3. In a man lift up the penis and hold it in a vertical position (Fig. 10.2a).
4. Begin to pass the catheter. Do not force it past any resistance; this may be a stricture and will only damage the urethra further and may create false passages.
5. When the catheter has advanced to the junction of the penile and membranous urethra at the level of the external sphincter, bring the penis down to lie horizontally while you advance the catheter through the prostatic urethra (Fig. 10.2b).
6. When urine begins to flow, inflate the balloon of the catheter.
7. Connect up the catheter collecting system.

NEEDLE CRICOTHYROIDOTOMY

It is unlikely that you will have to perform this procedure but, if required, it could save a life.

Indications

- Acute airway obstruction and inability to intubate
- A useful technique in emergency situations to provide oxygen until a definitive airway is placed.

You will need

- A 14-gauge needle and a syringe
- Antiseptic swabs
- Oxygen tubing with a hole cut towards the end.

Procedure

1. Palpate the cricothyroid membrane.
2. Insert the needle with the syringe at a 45° angle caudally until you aspirate air.
3. Connect with the oxygen tubing.
4. Intermittent ventilation is given by occluding the side hole in the tube for 1 s and releasing it for 4 s.

SUPRAPUBIC CATHETERIZATION

Indication

- This can only be done on a patient with retention and an enlarged, tense bladder.

You will need

- Sterile dressing pack, antiseptic solution, 20 ml of 1% lignocaine, a scalpel blade and a strong silk/nylon suture on a cutting needle
- A prepacked suprapubic catheter set
- An assistant.

Procedure

1. Explain the procedure to the patient.
2. Position the patient supine.
3. Clean the suprapubic skin and inject the local anaesthetic into the midline 3–4 cm above the symphysis pubis (Fig. 10.3a). Continue injecting through all layers until you withdraw urine.
4. Make a 1 cm incision in the skin at the site of injection of local anaesthetic.

5. Take the suprapubic catheter with the needle trocar in place and gently push it through the incision and on through the midline layers until you enter the bladder with a 'give' (Fig. 10.3b).
6. Withdraw the trocar and check to see that urine flows freely from the catheter.
7. Inflate the balloon on the catheter and suture the catheter to the skin.
8. Connect the catheter to the collecting system.

(a)

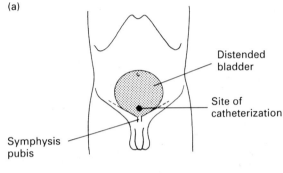

Distended bladder

Site of catheterization

Symphysis pubis

(b)

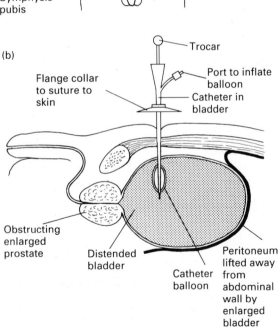

Trocar

Port to inflate balloon

Flange collar to suture to skin

Catheter in bladder

Obstructing enlarged prostate

Distended bladder

Catheter balloon

Peritoneum lifted away from abdominal wall by enlarged bladder

Fig. 10.3 Suprapubic catheterization. (a) Site; (b) insertion.

CENTRAL VENOUS CATHETERIZATION

Indications

- Central venous pressure monitoring
- Parenteral nutrition
- Inotrope (dopamine/dobutamine) support
- Cytotoxic chemotherapy
- Regular intravenous access if the peripheral veins are damaged.

You will need

- Sterile gloves and gown
- An appropriate commercially available central venous catheterization set, which should include:
  - 10–12 ml syringe with large-bore needle
  - A floppy-ended guidewire
  - Central venous catheter, to place over the guidewire (Seldinger technique)
- A 500 ml bag of normal saline, connected to a giving set and run through
- A sterile trolley laid out with a dressing pack and antiseptic
- Local anaesthetic (10 ml of 1% lignocaine)
- An assistant
- The patient placed on a bed with the capability of being tilted head down.

Procedure

1. With the patient lying supine on the bed, tilt the bed head down to cause venous engorgement of the great veins of the neck and upper chest. Paint the skin with antiseptic and infiltrate the site of puncture with local anaesthetic (Fig. 10.4):
   - *Internal jugular vein*: lateral to the carotid pulse at the level of the thyroid cartilage
   - *Subclavian vein*: junction of medial and middle third of the underside of the clavicle.
2. Now cannulate the vein using the needle and syringe:
   - *Internal jugular vein*: tilt the patient's head away from the side you are working on and guard the carotid artery with the fingers of one hand. Insert the needle slowly at an angle of 45° to the skin and aim towards the ipsilateral superior iliac spine (nipple in males). Gently aspirate as you advance and withdraw venous blood as you enter the vein
   - *Subclavian vein*: advance the needle with the bevel of the syringe passing under and against the lower border of the calvicle (Fig. 10.5a) and aiming at the region immediately behind the sternoclavicular joint, until you

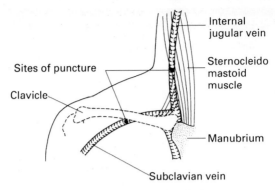

Fig. 10.4 Sites of central venous catheterization.

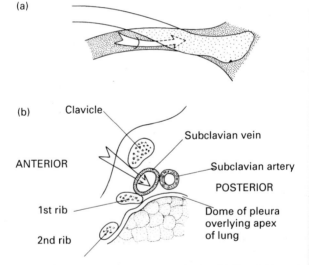

Fig. 10.5 Subclavian venous catheterization. (a) Site of skin entry and direction of needle under and against the undersurface of the junction of the medial and middle thirds of the clavicle; (b) cross-sectional view to show 'trajectory' of needle into subclavian vein. Note the proximity of the subclavian artery (behind) and the apex of the lung beneath the dome of the pleura (above).

withdraw venous blood: the confluence of the subclavian vein and the internal jugular vein (Fig. 10.5b).

3. In both cases, disconnect the syringe from the needle, beware the backflow of blood, and pass the Seldinger guidewire, *floppy-end first*, down the needle bore. If you have fluoroscopy screening available, it is worthwhile checking the position of the wire in the right atrium at this stage.

4. Remove the needle and slide the central venous cannula over the guidewire. Once in place, remove the guidewire, aspirate the cannula to check the easy flow of blood and connect the giving set to the cannula. Run through some saline to wash out any blood in the cannula. Suture the line in place and apply adhesive dressings to the entry site.

5. Check the position of the line and exclude a pneumothorax with a CXR.

6. Set up a central venous manometer and read the central venous pressure (Fig. 10.6).

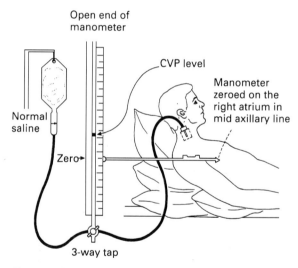

Fig. 10.6   Recording the central venous pressure.

> **Tips and problems**
>
> *Cardiac arrhythmias*: arise if the line is against the heart wall, and you should withdraw the line slightly.
>
> *Beware air embolism*: this is lethal. Check the tightness and seal of all your connections.
>
> *Pneumothorax*: always get a post-procedure CXR.
>
> *Clotting disorders*: this is a job for the experienced, not the beginner!
>
> *Infection*: suspect the central line in all patients who spike a pyrexia with a central line in place. Whenever the line has to be removed, always send the tip for microscopy, culture and sensitivity. If a line has to be removed because of sepsis, it may be possible to 'rail-road' a new cannula over a guidewire placed through the original cannula before it is removed.
>
> *Blocked cannula*: gently inject 10–20 ml of normal saline. If this fails, then it is safer to replace the cannula.
>
> *Hitting the carotid artery*: don't panic! Apply strong pressure for 5–10 min.

CARE OF CENTRAL VENOUS LINES

All central venous lines are a potential source of infection but this is of especial importance with long-term lines (Hickman or Nutricath) used for feeding.

Although nursing staff care for the day-to-day use of these lines it is not unusual for you to be asked to either flush these lines or to give i.v. antibiotics via them (this should be avoided if at all possible). It is very important that you can do this properly.

Here is a basic outline of how to disconnect a feeding line and flush it with heparin; the same technique applies to giving antibiotics.

You will need

- Sterile gloves ×2
- Dressing pack containing a Gallipot, sterile towels, gauze swabs ×5
- Vial of heparin (1000 units/ml)
- A 2 ml syringe and a green needle
- Tape
- Hydrex solution
- Assistant.

Procedure

1. Wash hands for >2 min using the Ayliffe technique.
2. Turn off infusion pump and clamp line.
3. Ask your assistant to open out the dressing pack, syringe and needle onto a sterile towel, then ask for Hydrex to be poured into the Gallipot.
4. Manusept your hands and put on two pairs of gloves.
5. Pick up a second towel and place it on the patient's chest as near as possible to the dressing surrounding the connector.
6. Remove the old dressing and discard without touching the connector; allow it to drop onto the second towel. Now remove your outer pair of gloves.
7. Using your assistant to hold the vial, first wipe the top with gauze soaked in Hydrex and then draw up 2.5 ml of heparin.
8. Using a piece of sterile gauze disconnect the old line and allow it to fall away from the patient, clear of your sterile field.
9. Using a swab dipped in Hydrex, wipe once around the bioconnector. Repeat to dry
10. Insert your syringe tightly into the connector; *do not use a needle*. Ask your assistant to unclamp the line and inject the heparin gently into it. Ask the assistant to clamp the line just before the syringe is empty. *Do not force the heparin into the line, as this can crack the surface covering.*
11. Place a gauze dressing around the connector wrapping it in tape. Finally secure the dressing to the patient's chest as close to the exit site as possible and with the connector facing upwards.
12. Dispose of your rubbish and sharps carefully.

ASPIRATION OF A PLEURAL EFFUSION

Indications

- Pleural effusion, either transudative or the result of a reactive exudate
- Early empyema, before organization.

You will need

- Sterile gloves
- Chest aspiration pack (containing sterile dressing pack, large syringe, long wide-bore needle (or green needle followed by a venflon), three-way tap and large jug)
- Local anaesthetic (20 ml of 1% lignocaine)
- Specimen bottles:
  - Biochemistry

- Microbiology
- Cytology
- An assistant.

Preparation

Position the patient, seated over a bedside table (Fig. 10.7a).
Get the patient to rest their face on a pillow.

Procedure

1. Percuss out the level of the effusion and confirm the side
   of the effusion.
2. Infiltrate the local anaesthetic into the 9th intercostal
   space near the posterior axillary line just below the scapula
   (Fig. 10.7b). Wait 5 min.

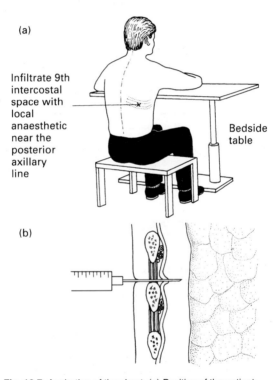

(a)

Infiltrate 9th
intercostal
space with
local
anaesthetic
near the
posterior
axillary
line

Bedside
table

(b)

Fig. 10.7 Aspiration of the chest. (a) Position of the patient;
(b) position of the aspirating needle placed over the rib (to avoid
the intercostal neurovascular bundle) and into the pleural
effusion.

3. Mount the three-way tap onto the syringe and attach the needle to the three-way tap.
4. Gently insert the needle through the anaesthetized skin and slide the needle *over* the 10th rib into the pleural space, so avoiding the 9th intercostal neurovascular bundle.
5. Aspirate the effusion, taking samples of the first aspirate for laboratory investigation. As the syringe fills, empty the contents via the three-way tap into the jug. Take about 1 litre of the effusion at each sitting, no more.
6. When finished, place a waterproof dressing over the site and obtain a CXR.

Tips and problems

Dry tap? May be an organized empyema. Get help.

Pneumothorax. Get help. It may be possible to aspirate the air but it is probably due to puncturing the lung and is better managed with a chest drain.

Unexpectedly very bloody aspirate. Get help. Have you punctured an intercostal vessel? Keep the patient on quarter-hourly observation for the next 3–4 h and repeat the CXR at this time.

INTERCOSTAL NERVE BLOCK

Indications

- Relief of pain due to broken ribs
- Post-thoracotomy analgesia.

You will need

- Sterile gloves
- A 20 ml syringe and 21-gauge (green) needle
- 20 ml of 1% marcaine
- Dressing pack and topical skin antiseptic.

Preparation

1. Position the patient as for a pleural aspiration (Fig. 10.7a).
2. Prep the skin:
   - *Broken ribs*: over the back of the chest, medial to the site(s) of fracture, always include the rib above and the rib below the broken rib(s)
   - *Post-thoracotomy*: over the back of the chest, medial to the posterior border of the scar (usually along the 6th rib), including the rib above and the rib below.

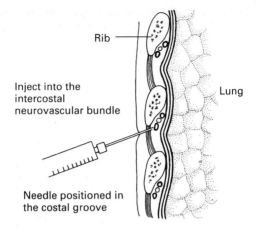

Rib

Inject into the
intercostal
neurovascular bundle

Lung

Needle positioned in
the costal groove

Fig. 10.8 Intercostal nerve block.

Procedure

1. Gently insert the needle of the syringe containing the
   marcaine down to the lower border of the rib overlying the
   intercostal nerve to be blocked.
2. Unlike a pleural aspiration, pass the needle immediately
   under the rib to lie adjacent to the neurovascular bundle
   (Fig. 10.8). Aspirate and, if no blood or air is drawn back,
   then infiltrate 3–5 ml of marcaine.
3. Repeat the procedure at the other sites.
4. Obtain a CXR to exclude a pneumothorax.

> **Tips and problems**
>
> If you draw blood or air, slowly withdraw the needle
> several millimetres and reaspirate.

SIMPLE AVULSION OF AN INGROWN TOE NAIL

Indication

- Ingrown great toe nail.

You will need

- Sterile heavy artery forceps and scalpel
- Tourniquet
- Dressing pack

- Local anaesthetic (51 ml of 2% *plain* lignocaine mixed with 5 ml of 0.5% marcaine) (do *not* use lignocaine with adrenaline on fingers and toes)
- 10 ml syringe and 23-gauge (blue) needle.

Procedure

1. Prep the forefoot with antiseptic and drape the foot to expose the great toe.
2. Infiltrate all four digital nerves of the toe with local anaesthetic (the two dorsal and two plantar nerves) by approaching them from the plantar surface at the sites shown (Fig. 10.9a). Wait 5 min.
3. Place the tourniquet around the proximal toe and make two small nicks down to the nail in the two corners of the nail fold (Fig. 10.9b).
4. Pass the heavy artery forceps down under the lateral border of the nail and grasp the nail. With a motion akin to that of opening a tin of sardines, avulse the nail by

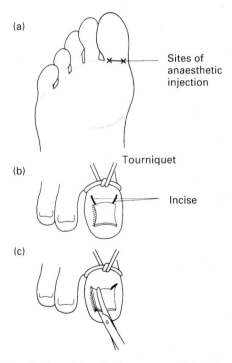

Fig. 10.9 Simple avulsion of an ingrown toe nail. (a) Sites of injection of anaesthetic; (b) site of incision; (c) avulsion.

rolling it out of its nailbed (Fig. 10.9c). Repeat this on the other side of the nail and remove the nail.
5. Dress the nailbed with paraffin gauze and remove the tourniquet. Dress the toe and forefoot in dressing gauze.
6. Advise the patient to rest at home with the foot elevated. This will lessen the pain.

Do not worry about the *initial bleeding*. Unless you have inadvertently operated on someone with a clotting disorder (call for help) the bleeding always settles.

Unanaesthetized toe: wait a bit longer; still unanaesthetized? Give more local anaesthetic.

EXCISION OF A SEBACEOUS CYST

Indication

- Sebaceous cyst.

You will need

- Minor operation set (essentially a scalpel, toothed forceps, needle holder, artery forceps)
- Local anaesthetic (10 ml of 1% lignocaine with 1 in 200 000 adrenaline)
- Antiseptic and sterile drapes
- 3/0 nylon/silk skin suture on a cutting needle.

Preparation

1. If the cyst(s) is/are on the scalp then cut away the overlying hair.
2. Prep the skin, and infiltrate the skin *surrounding* the cyst with local anaesthetic (Fig. 10.10a). If you infiltrate into the cyst, all that happens is that the anaesthetic will come squirting out of the punctum into your eye. What's more, it will smell of old sebum! Wait 5 min.

Procedure

1. Incise the skin overlying the cyst in an ellipse (Fig. 10.10b) down to the white capsule of the cyst.
2. Insert the artery forceps between the skin and capsule of the cyst and open them to establish a tissue plane (Fig. 10.10c). Continue all around the cyst.
3. Gently lift the cyst out, dividing any remaining strands of fibrous tissue (Fig. 10.10d). Crush any small vessels with the artery forceps.

4. Close the skin with interrupted sutures (Fig. 10.10e). Pick up the floor of the cyst with each stitch.
5. Remove the sutures 1 week later.

> **Tips and problems**
>
> *Infected sebaceous cyst*: treat with antibiotics (flucloxacillin) and excise when infection resolves.
>
> *Capsule bursts during excision*: do not just simply drain the cyst; it will recur. Excise the capsule.

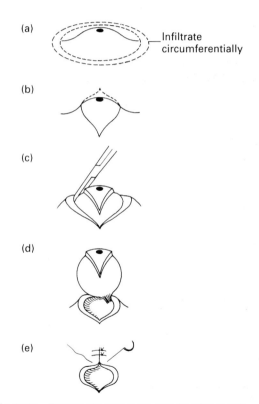

Fig. 10.10 Excision of a sebaceous cyst. (a) Infiltrate with anaesthetic; (b) incise an ellipse of overlying skin; (c) pass blunt forceps under skin, open to create space in tissue plane around the cyst and lift out cyst; (d) divide remaining strands of fibrous tissue; (e) close using interrupted sutures.

EXCISION OF A SKIN PAPILLOMA/LESION

Indication

- Excision or biopsy of an unwanted skin lesion.

You will need

As for a sebaceous cyst (see page 188).

Preparation

As for a sebaceous cyst (see page 188) (Fig. 10.11a).

Procedure

1. Incise the skin around the lesion in an elliptical manner in the direction of adjacent skin creases (Fig. 10.11b).
2. Excise the lesion and *send it for histological examination*.
3. Close the skin with interrupted sutures (Fig. 10.11c).
4. Remove sutures 1 week later.

> **Tips and problems**
>
> *Excessive bleeding*: apply pressure and call for help.
>
> *Suspicion of malignancy?* Be sure to excise the lesion with a reasonable 5–10 mm margin.

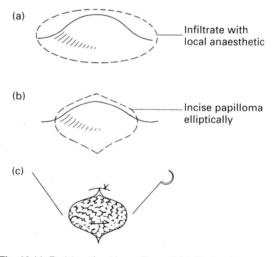

(a) ———— Infiltrate with local anaesthetic

(b) ———— Incise papilloma elliptically

(c)

Fig. 10.11 Excision of a skin papilloma. (a) Infiltrate with anaesthetic; (b) incise papilloma elliptically; (c) close with interrupted sutures.

EXCISION OF A SUBCUTANEOUS LIPOMA

Indication

- Troublesome subcutaneous lipoma in a patient who cannot be persuaded to leave it alone.

You will need

As for a sebaceous cyst (see page 188).

Preparation

As for a sebaceous cyst (see page 188) (Fig. 10.12a).

Procedure

1. Incise the overlying skin in the direction of the adjacent skin creases and continue down to the capsule of the lipoma (Fig. 10.12b).
2. Break down any bands that lie over the lipoma, loculating and entrapping it.
3. Gently remove the lipoma using a combination of traction and external pressure, like shelling out a pea from a pod (Fig. 10.12c). *Send the specimen for histological examination.*
4. Close the skin with interrupted sutures, picking up the base of the wound to help haemostasis (Fig. 10.12d).
5. Remove sutures after 1 week.

> **Tips and problems**
>
> *Excessive bleeding?* Apply pressure for 5–10 min. If bleeding stops, fine, close and apply a pressure dressing. If still bleeding, call for help.
>
> *Doesn't look yellow and fatty?* Is it a lymph node or a subcutaneous metastasis? Get help.

PARACENTESIS ABDOMINIS

Indications

- Diagnostic tap of ascites
- Therapeutic tap of ascites to relieve respiratory embarrassment
- Abdominal trauma: looking for free blood (however, this technique is not as accurate as peritoneal lavage (see page 130), which should be done by your Registrar).

You will need

- Minor dressing pack

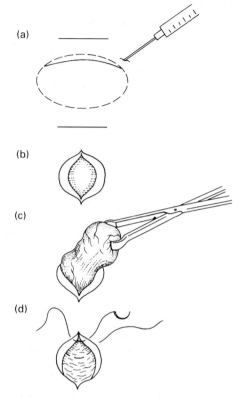

Fig. 10.12 Excision of a subcutaneous lipoma. (a) Infiltrate the skin with anaesthetic; (b) incise the skin down to the lipoma capsule; (c) withdraw the lipoma, breaking down any adhesions; (d) close with interrupted mattress sutures, taking in all layers including the base of the cavity.

- Antiseptic
- Local anaestheitic (10 ml of 1% lignocaine)
- 20 ml syringe and 21-gauge (green) needle for a diagnostic tap
- 60 ml syringe and 16-gauge needle, and a three-way tap if for a therapeutic tap (see aspirating a pleural effusion, page 183)
- Specimen bottles for:
  – Biochemistry (protein content)
  – Microbiology
  – Cytology
- An assistant is useful but not essential for a diagnostic tap.

Preparation

1. Position the patient in as comfortable a supine position as they can manage.
2. Percuss out the position of the ascites and prep the skin where the precussion note is dull. If the tap is looking for blood within the peritoneum after trauma, then prep the skin in all four quadrants of the abdomen (four-quadrant tap).
3. Infiltrate the sites of the tap down to, and including, the peritoneum with local anaesthetic.

Procedure

1. Pass the needle through the abdominal wall, gently aspirating as you go. As you enter the peritoneal cavity you will draw back straw-coloured fluid if you find ascites. Send samples for laboratory investigation.
2. If you are draining ascites, then proceed to aspirate the fluid as for a pleural effusion (see page 183). If following trauma, then suspect a ruptured abdominal viscus if you draw back deeply blood-stained fluid.
3. Withdraw the needle and dress the wound.

Tips and problems

Only get out 'so much' and then it stops: the ascitic collection may be loculated. Try again under ultrasound control.

Bloody tap in one quadrant only in a patient who may have only had minimal trauma and is haemodynamically stable: you may have hit a blood vessel, particularly an epigastric. You should call for help and get your Registrar to perform a peritoneal lavage.

STOMA CARE

You will not normally be involved in stoma care as there is usually a specialist nurse available who can do this and they will always know more than you do. If there isn't a specialist nurse, one of the Ward Sisters who deals with patients undergoing operations that result in stomas will almost certainly have some expertise. Failing this, all of the companies that produce stoma products have specialists who will advise in difficult situations. So, if you are asked to deal with a problem, e.g. a badly fitting stoma, and you can't get anybody to sort it out, ring the company that manufactures the product. There are also a few tips worth pointing out.

- *Badly fitting stoma*. This can often be dealt with by filling up the crevices (where scarring has led to irregular skin and the stomas do not fit properly) with some sort of gum.

- *Stoma leakage.* Different kinds of gums can be used and specialist adhesives may help to deal with this.
- *Prolapsed stoma (particularly colostomy).* These can be a real problem and often require major surgery to correct them. You will not be involved in this and the main point is *not* to tell patients that they should have revisional surgery without being sure that they are suitable for it.
- *Para-colostomy hernia.* This can become quite painful and you may worry that herniae are strangulated. Occasionally they do strangulate but more often they are simply distended with faeces and a small enema into the colostomy will do the trick. Do not forget that you can examine a colostomy exactly as you would an anal canal, including doing a digital examination if need be.
- The *colour of colostomies* after operation is often a cause of concern and you may be called to the ward to pass judgement. The main problem is that a colostomy often looks rather bruised and the nurses may be worried that it is in fact ischaemic.
    - If the discolouration is localized, with some of the circumference pink, then don't worry. Even if there is an ischaemic area it will be localized.
    - If the whole circumsference looks bluey-black, then just pass a proctoscope or sigmoidoscope (see page 199) gently into the outer part of the colostomy and see if 1 cm or so back is pink. If so, then again you need not worry even if the tip is necrotic – it should not retract. However, this is worth pointing out to the Surgeon concerned. If there is deeper ischaemia, then there may be local peritonism and this can be elicited clinically. In the absence of peritonism, providing there is continuity, the management is usually conservative but in any case let your seniors know.

ENT

There are two procedures you need to know about:

- How to deal with epistaxis
- How to remove a foreign body from the nose or ear.

Epistaxis

The vast majority of cases will stop spontaneously. The usual treatment is to place the patient in the sitting position, leaning forward with a bowl underneath their face. Get them to hold the bridge of their nose but not to swallow or do anything else. Blood and saliva should be allowed to run into the bowl and sooner or later it should stop.

Obviously swallowing and blowing the nose will dislodge clots and these reactions should be resisted for as long as possible to ensure haemostasis. In the unusual circumstance that this does not work it may be necessary to pack the offending nostril. This is extremely uncomfortable for the patient and usually requires local analgesia of some kind. The procedure itself, however, is straightforward and simply entails packing ribbon gauze with long forceps into the nasal cavity until the bleeding has arrested. Very occasionally the retropharyngeal space may need to be packed and in this case a soft catheter is passed along the floor of the nasal cavity into the pharynx and then into the back of the throat. It is important not to get bitten while retrieving the end of the catheter! The catheter can then be used to feed a pack into the space. It is unlikely though that a House Surgeon inexperienced in this technique will be called upon to practise it.

Foreign bodies

The important thing about foreign bodies is not to make the situation worse and this means *not* pushing the foreign body any further into the nose or ear. Special forceps exist for removing foreign bodies, but the easiest way to do it, providing you can see the foreign body directly, is to apply a blob of superglue or impact adhesive to the end of an orange stick or matchstick and carefully apply it to the foreign body, wait for it to set and then pull the foreign body out. Whatever you do *don't* stick the superglue to the patient's skin because you will get little gratitude for supergluing a piece of wood to the inside of somebody's nose or ear!

APPLICATION OF TRACTION FOR ORTHOPAEDIC USE

Traction can seem complicated but is in fact simple. Its aims are to provide a distracting force sufficient to overcome the tendency of muscles to cause overlap of fractured bone ends and to adjust the direction of the force in such a way that the ends of the bone will unite in the correct position. For practical purposes, traction is appropriate for injuries to the long bones of the lower limb.

Femoral fracture

A Thomas frame is usually used, which fits over the leg and has pulleys on the lower end to allow the distracting force to be placed. Traction may be applied temporarily using bandage or adhesive tape applied to the lower leg, but usually a pin is passed through the tibial condyles to allow long-term traction. The orientation of the lower leg, which is flexed at approximately 15° at the knee, together with the direction of the traction adjusted by varying the degree of adduction and abduction at the hip, will bring the orientation of the two ends of the femur into line. X-rays are taken in position to ensure that this is the case. If the ends of the bone overlap, the tractive force is insufficient and more weight should be added. If the bones are parted then the force is excessive and weight should be removed.

Tibial fractures

A similar system is employed but here a pin is passed through the calcaneum. The position of this bone is harder to adjust and great care must be taken with both angle and circular orientation. Small variations in femoral alignment can be corrected at the hip, which is a ball and socket joint and capable of movement in any direction. If there is inversion or eversion of the foot due to faulty setting of a tibial fracture, permanent disability is likely as the knee, a hinge joint, cannot account for this. A similar principle applies to the adjustment of weight.

Humeral fractures

Traction is also occasionally applied to fractures of the head and shaft of the humerus. A collar and cuff sling is applied to the wrist and the tractive force in this case is provided by the weight of the arm. Because the shoulder is a ball and socket joint it can, as the hip does, overcome small variations in the angle set by the humerus and the positioning is not quite so critical.

Back injuries

Traction applied to the treatment of back injuries is usually specifically for injuries of the neck, where Crutchfield tongs are usually placed in the outer table of the skull, and weight is applied to distract the cervical spine. The patient is usually placed on a bed sloping downwards at about $15°$ so that the weight of their body provides counter-traction. The important point is to tighten the tongs gradually, week-by-week, otherwise they will suddenly disconnect, leading at least to a painful surprise for the patient and possibly to dislocation of the neck.

Traction for the rest of the spine is usually employed only in non-specific types of back pain and tends to be applied as seems appropriate for the individual.

APPLICATION OF PLASTER

Application or adjustment of plaster of Paris is occasionally asked of the House Surgeon and some outlines on how to do this are of use.

If the plaster is to be applied to hold a fractured bone in position this may be the end of a manipulation under anaesthesia in theatre or in the A & E Department. More often, however, you may be asked to change plasters where the position is relatively stable. In either case adequate support must be given to the limb in question.

Removal of plaster is usually straightforward using the plaster saw, which oscillates and therefore does not cut the skin which can move with it. If the saw is dragged quickly along the skin it will, however, cut and the blade should therefore be rolled along the plaster as it cuts. Properly guarded scissors or shears should be used to cut the deeper layer so as to avoid the tip of the instrument digging into the skin.

Although it is possible to apply plaster of Paris on your own, it is of very considerable advantage to have an assistant.

Preparation

1. The area of application must be suitable to allow water and plaster to be splashed on it and the patient should also be dressed suitably so that their clothing is not spoiled by plaster dust or splashes of liquid plaster. Expose the area where the plaster is to be applied together with the adjacent area and apply towelling or waterproof drapes to protect the rest of the patient.
2. Prepare a bowl of water and the number of plaster bandages that you think you will require. These should be assembled on a trolley so that you can apply the plasters without having to take off their wrappings once your hands are wet.

> **Remember**
>
> The plaster can be quite irritant to the skin.

Procedure

1. Get your assistant to support the limb distally and apply the woollen bandage so that it is snug but not tight. Note that one of the principal sources of overtight plasters is the wool rather than the plaster itself.
2. Once the wool has been applied, and this should be done exactly as for a normal bandage, take the first plaster bandage, emerse it in water and allow the bubbles to escape from between the rolls. Remove from the water, squeeze once and apply so that the plaster bandage is not loose and yet not overly tight. Bandages should be overlapped slightly, as with any bandage, but not wound round and round.
3. If extra thickness is required, further layers of bandage should be applied over the first, ideally before the first has dried because the bandages will bind together much better if both are wet.

4. When the final bandage has been applied and the application of the cast is complete, wet both hands and wash off any plaster that may be beginning to dry on them and then, with wet hands, rub gently over the plaster. This will give it a pleasing smooth appearance and, more importantly, allow you to mould it to fit before it sets fully.

5. As the plaster begins to set you will feel it increase in temperature and once it has started to get hot it will be set within a few minutes. However, initially it will be very soft and this is the main time when plasters crack. Therefore, tell the patient not to stretch the plaster for at least half an hour and that it will not reach full strength for 24 h, by which time it will be dry through. (This applies to plaster of Paris – some of the modern synthetic plasters will set almost immediately to their full strength.)

6. When the plaster has been applied it is usual to split it if the limb has recently been broken, i.e. if this is the first application of plaster. To do this it is usually necessary to use plaster shears because the plaster saw will not cut damp plaster very effectively. If the plaster is being split, either as part of its initial application or because the patient complains of symptoms of plaster tightness, i.e. those of pressure, then the plaster must be split all the way to the skin. If the bandage is left intact the pressure may

Remember

Application of plaster is an art and it may be that the first few will need to be changed until the appropriate application is achieved.

Tips and problems

The *temperature of the water* in which the plaster of Paris is soaked will determine the speed at which the plaster sets, so that if you are not very experienced cool water is best since this will allow the most time for adjustment. On the other hand, the longer the time the greater the chance that the patient will move and the plaster, once cracked, will never be fully strong. Always use cold water to apply synthetic plaster, otherwise the plaster is hard before you have finished the roll. A dent in a synthetic plaster or a sharp edge by lack of enough wool padding is unforgiving and will need readjustment.

It is absolutely vital that no patient who complains of *an overly tight plaster* is ignored, since disastrous consequences of ischaemia to muscle, nerve damage or skin sores may develop.

not be relieved. It is particularly important to avoid pressure where nerves run between skin and bone since neural damage is most likely at these sites, the classical area being below-knee plasters which come too close to the knee. If a plaster is found to be too tight at one pressure point it is usually possible either to use some form of plaster tong or cutter to soften it locally or simply to break it with the thumbs in the area of tightness without having to change the whole plaster.

BALLOON TAMPONADE FOR VARICEAL BLEEDING

This will not usually fall to the House Surgeon. However, an understanding of the principles is useful and you may find yourself in the situation of being the only person around when a patient with a Sengstaken-Blakemore tube in place gets into difficulties.

The tube has four channels and two balloons (Fig. 10.13a). The first channel aspirates the stomach below the gastric balloon; the second is for the gastric balloon; the third controls the oesophageal balloon; and the fourth channel is to aspirate oesophageal contents and secretions above the oesophageal balloon.

Procedure

1. The patient is positioned head down to reduce the chances of aspiration of gastric contents during intubation.
2. The tube is passed orally; once in place the *gastric* balloon is inflated to a pressure of 60 mmHg and the tube then pulled back to anchor the balloon against the cardia.
3. The *oesophageal* balloon is then inflated to a pressure of 40–50 mmHg (Fig. 10.13b). Tension on the tube is achieved by taping a tongue depressor at right angles to the tube and against the mouth.
4. Aspirate both the *gastric* and *oesophageal* balloons every 30 min and every hour let the *oesophageal* balloon down to reduce the chances of mucosal ulceration.

PROCTOSCOPY AND SIGMOIDOSCOPY

You will probably not be asked to undertake these procedures. However, mastering the technique may be a useful addition to the armamentarium of your capabilities.

Indications

- Examination of all perianal symptoms, including rectal bleeding and altered bowel habit

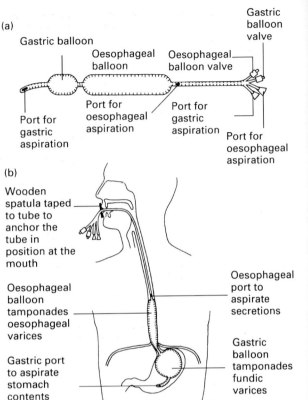

(a)

Gastric balloon

Oesophageal balloon

Oesophageal balloon valve

Gastric balloon valve

Port for gastric aspiration

Port for oesophageal aspiration

Port for gastric aspiration

Port for oesophageal aspiration

(b)

Wooden spatula taped to tube to anchor the tube in position at the mouth

Oesophageal balloon tamponades oesophageal varices

Gastric port to aspirate stomach contents

Oesophageal port to aspirate secretions

Gastric balloon tamponades fundic varices

Fig. 10.13 (a) The four channels and two balloons of the Sengstaken–Blakemore tube; (b) balloons in position and inflated.

- Treatment of haemorrhoids
- Should be done routinely before every barium enema.

You will need

- A proctoscope
- A sigmoidoscope
- A light source
- Lubricating jelly
- Gauze swabs
- An assistant.

In addition, you may need a glass syringe and haemorrhoid

needle with 10 ml of phenol in almond oil or a Barron's band applicator to deal with piles. If investigating the cause of rectal bleeding you will need biopsy forceps and a sterile pot with formalin.

Preparation

1. Position the patient on the couch in the left lateral position.
2. Reassure the patient strongly.
3. Carefully examine the external anal canal and perform a gentle rectal examination. Points to note are:
   – Pain and tenderness
   – Tumours both within the anus and rectum and compressing the rectum extrinsically
   – Boggy mass in the pelvis suggestive of a pelvic collection.

Procedure

Proctoscopy

Perform this first. It will examine the anal canal and not the rectum.

1. With the trocar in place, lubricate the proctoscope and connect it to the light source.
2. Gently insert the instrument in a direction aimed at the umbilicus, passing it up to the hilt.
3. Remove the trocar.
4. Now examine the rectal mucosa which pouts into the opening of the scope. The structures/pathologies to note are:
   – Rectal mucosa
   – Dentate line
   – Anal mucosa
   – Vascular anal cushions
   – Haemorrhoids at 4, 7 and 11 o'clock
   – Fissure in ano lying either at 12 or 6 o'clock
   – Opening of a fistula
   – Anal skin tags.
5. Gently and slowly withdraw the scope noting the transition from rectal to anal mucosa as you pass the dentate line.

Injecting of piles

1. Visualize the uppermost point of the haemorrhoid *above* the dentate line (Fig. 10.14a).
2. Inject the phenol and almond oil (2–5 ml) into the rectal mucosa at this point, causing a mucosal blister (Fig. 10.14b).
3. Withdraw the needle and inject the other piles.

Banding of piles

1. Visualize the whole pile bulging into the proctoscope (Fig. 10.14a).

2. Place the pile-grasping forceps through the band applicator (Fig. 10.14c).
3. Grasp the pile and pass the band applicator up over the pile as you draw it down.
4. Place the band applicators *above* the dentate line and release the band (Fig. 10.14c).

Never band more than two piles at one session.

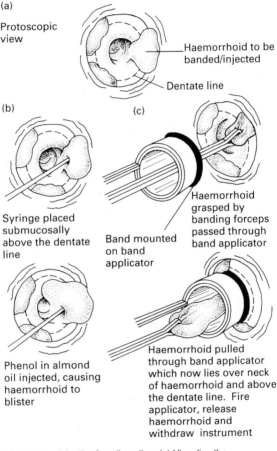

(a)

Protoscopic view

Haemorrhoid to be banded/injected

Dentate line

(b)   (c)

Syringe placed submucosally above the dentate line

Band mounted on band applicator

Haemorrhoid grasped by banding forceps passed through band applicator

Phenol in almond oil injected, causing haemorrhoid to blister

Haemorrhoid pulled through band applicator which now lies over neck of haemorrhoid and above the dentate line. Fire applicator, release haemorrhoid and withdraw instrument

Fig. 10.14 Injecting/banding piles. (a) Visualize the haemorrhoid/pile; (b) injecting piles; (c) banding piles.

Sigmoidoscopy

Warn the patient that this will be an uncomfortable and embarrassing procedure, but despite this it will not be dangerous.

Procedure

1. Gently pass the lubricated sigmoidoscope with trocar in place into the anal canal.
2. Remove the trocar and attach the eyepiece with insufflator.
3. Gently begin to inflate the rectum while visualizing the rectal mucosa. As a clear passage opens up, advance the sigmoidoscope into the space. *Never* force the scope blindly against the mucosa. Negotiate the sigmoidoscope past the valves of Houston to reach the rectosigmoid junction. You can go *no* further.
4. Note:
   – Rectal mucosa: colour, consistency, contact bleeding
   – Polyps and tumours
   – Extrinsic compression
   – Diverticulae/fistulae
   – Stool: colour, consistency.

Biopsy of granular mucosa (contact bleeding) or tumour

1. Use the sigmoidoscopy biopsy forceps.
2. Take several pieces of tumour or mucosa.
3. Place them immediately in formalin:
   – In the case of mucosa, try to place them mucosal surface up on a piece of blotting paper before placing them in formalin. This will orientate the Histopathologist.
4. Warn the patient that they will bleed for a time.

INSERTION AND MANAGEMENT OF A CHEST DRAIN

Indications

- Pneumothorax
- Haemothorax
- Post-thoracotomy.

You will need

- Sterile gloves and gown
- Dressing pack (antiseptic, scalpel, artery forceps, strong 0 or 1 nylon or silk suture)
- Chest drain cannula; discard the trocar that comes with it
- Chest drain bottle filled with 300 ml of sterile water to the zero mark
- Local anaesthetic (20 ml of 1% lignocaine), syringe and green needle
- Dressings and adhesive plastic tape
- An assistant.

Procedure

1. Strongly reassure the patient.
2. Determine the site of drainage:
   - 2nd/3rd intercostal space in the mid-clavicular line
     (Fig. 10.15). This site is strongly favoured by physicians.
     It is reasonable if all you want to evacuate is air but as
     useful as a chocolate teapot if you want to drain fluid,
     particularly blood!
   - 5th intercostal space in the mid-axillary line (this is at
     the level of the nipple)
   - 8th or 9th intercostal space in the mid-axillary line
     (Fig. 10.15). Much more useful and much favoured by
     Surgeons. You must be careful to remember the great
     solid viscera of the abdomen lie immediately below the
     diaphragm at these points, i.e. the liver and the spleen.
3. Infiltrate the site of drain insertion with local anaesthetic,
   down through the intercostal space and including the
   parietal pleura (Fig. 10.16a). Wait 5 min.
4. Make a 2 cm skin incision in the line of the intercostal
   space and deepen to muscle. Place a mattress suture in the
   middle of your incision with a strong 0 or 1 nylon and tape
   both ends to the skin. After taking the drain out, this will
   give a much neater scar than the more commonly used
   pursestring suture (especially the female patient will be
   grateful for this).
5. Insert the sinus forceps or artery clip deep into the incision
   and through the intercostal muscle fibres. Open the
   forceps to spread the fibres apart (Fig. 10.16b). Open the
   pleura with a scalpel under direct vision. Gently push the
   forceps through the parietal pleura.
6. Pass the chest drain cannula gently down through the
   incision and, without any trocar, into the pleural space
   (Fig. 10.16c). This should lead to an escape of blood
   and/or air. Direct into the required position and suture the

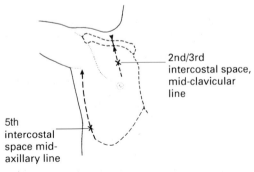

2nd/3rd
intercostal space,
mid-clavicular
line

5th
intercostal
space mid-
axillary line

Fig. 10.15 Positions for insertion of a chest drain.

(a)

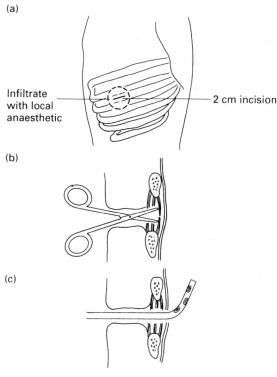

Infiltrate with local anaesthetic

2 cm incision

(b)

(c)

Fig. 10.16 Placing a chest drain. (a) Infiltrate with local anaesthetic and make an incision; (b) insert forceps and spread fibres; (c) introduce chest drain cannula into pleural cavity.

    drain in place and connect the chest drain cannula to the arm of the underwater seal, which extends below the water level of the chest drain bottle (Fig. 10.17).

7. Always obtain a CXR immediately after insertion of a chest drain:
 – To check the position of the drain and make sure all the side holes of the drain are *within* the pleural cavity
 – To check that the lung has reinflated.
8. Remove the tube when it is not draining any more:
 – There is no further bubbling
 – Fluid drainage is <100 ml per day
 – The lung is inflated on the CXR.

    Give parenteral analgesia before removal of the drain. Ask the patient to do a Valsalva manoeuvre (exercise first), pull out

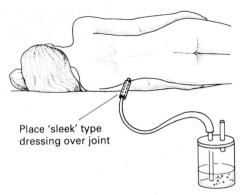

Place 'sleek' type
dressing over joint

Connect to long arm
of underwater seal

Fig. 10.17 Chest drain connected to underwater seal.

the drain and tie the mattress suture in one go. Take a CXR immediately after removal to confirm you didn't cause a pneumothorax.

Tips and problems

Ensure that the *water level* in the drainage tube is held above that of the rest of the water in the bottle and swings on respiration and coughing. If the water column is not swinging then either your drain tube is not in the pleural space or it is blocked.

Persistent bubbling means there is a broncho-pleural fistula. Place the drain on a low suction pressure Robert's pump at a pressure of 5 cm H_2O.

Keep two clamps beside the patient. *Clamp* the tube if the patient is being moved.

11

Useful drugs

Within 5 min of starting your first house job a drug card will be thrust into your hand and you will be asked to prescribe something for Mr Strainalots bowels. Don't panic, follow the guidelines in this chapter and you'll soon be doing it in your sleep.

Each hospital will have its own form of drug card, but essentially they all contain three sections:

- prn medication: those drugs to be given as and when required, e.g. analgesia
- Regular medication: those drugs that are to be given at a set time each day, e.g. antihypertensives
- One-off drugs: as the name suggests, individual doses of a drug to be given only once, e.g. enemas.

Prescribing a drug in any section involves the following:

1. The generic name, e.g. omeprazole not Losec (the trade name)
2. The dose, including the units
3. Route of administration, e.g. p.o., i.v., p.r. (see front of book for abbreviations)
4. Times for administration: use 24-hour clock (regular and one-off drugs only)
5. Frequency and maximum dose in 24 h (prn drugs only)
6. Your signature and date for starting medication.

Tips for prescribing

- The most important thing to remember when prescribing is that if you have any doubt about the dose, side-effects, contraindications or interactions *refer to the BNF or your hospital formulary.*
- Write clearly, especially the dose and units – mg and mcg look very alike when scrawled in a hurry; if necessary, write out micrograms. Doctors have been successfully sued in the past when the wrong dose of a drug has been given because the nurse couldn't read the prescription properly!
- When admitting a patient be sure to write up all their regular medication plus any new medication you are starting. It you feel a patient may possible need analgesia or an antiemetic in the future it is a good idea to write these up on a prn basis as it may save you a journey from your bed in the middle of the night.

Verbal prescribing

Although increasingly frowned upon by Trusts, some nursing staff are still prepared to give simple medication or fluids on your verbal authorization. This is very useful if a patient has a headache in the middle of the night. The nurse who does this is responsible for any consequences until you sign for the drug so you must remember to sign the prescription form as soon as possible. If a nurse refuses to give unprescribed medication it is your responsibility not hers (remember nurses can be struck off far more easily than doctors!).

Drug monitoring

Some drugs in common use require regular monitoring to check that blood concentration is in the therapeutic range. These include digoxin, gentamicin, phenytoin, lithium and amiodarone. Each drug differs in the time that the blood needs to be taken and what colour tube it needs to be sent in, so liaise with your hospital's clinical chemistry lab for details.

Intravenous drugs

More and more hospitals are training nursing staff to give common i.v. medication such as antibiotics; however, if this is not the case in your hospital or for some less common drugs, you will be asked to give them. Before giving an i.v. drug you need to ask whether the patient really requires the drug i.v. (they are often very expensive as well as being time-consuming), what the drug and dose are and how you are going to give the drug. Check the BNF to see if the drug can be given directly or whether it needs to be given as an infusion over a longer period of time. If it is to be given as an infusion, find out from the BNF what it can be mixed with (usually normal saline or 5% dextrose) and then make up the bag with a nurse to check the dose, making sure you clearly label the bag with what you have put in it and how quickly it should be given. Find out from a senior nurse how to set up an infusion pump (it's not difficult) as you may be asked to do this as well. Remember to check the infusion against the patient's drug chart and identification bracelet (or ask them who they are).

Controlled drugs

In order to send a patient home with a supply of a controlled drug you will be asked to fill in a special prescription form. Legally this must be completed in a very particular way otherwise it will be rejected by pharmacy:

- Write the whole prescription in your own handwriting and in pen
- Fill in all sections including the patient's name and address, and the date
- Use the drug's generic name
- Write the daily dose of the drug and its form, e.g. tablets, capsules, liquid
- Write the total number of dose units to be prescribed in both numbers and letters, e.g. 5 days supply of MST 120 mg b.d. would be prescribed as 20 (twenty) 60 mg tablets.

Owing to geographical differences in bacterial sensitivities, each hospital has its own antibiotic policy. This section therefore deals with general principles of antibiotic prescribing rather than specific drugs. Consult your hospital formulary for individual drugs and doses.

Antibiotics selectively kill organisms that are sensitive to them. As a result, if used for prolonged periods resistant organisms may emerge. Therefore, antibiotics should be used carefully and only with positive indications.

Usually a clinical diagnosis of bacterial infection is made before bacteriological results are available and antibiotics are commenced on a best-guess basis; continuation of a 'full course' of these antibiotics is dependent upon bacteriological substantiation of this infection.

Therapeutic recommendations for starting antibiotics can be found in your hospital formulary.

Antibiotics should *always* be stopped if an organism is demonstrated to be resistant to them and only in a few cases should any therapeutic course of antibiotics exceed 7 days.

Septicaemia

Diagnosis

- Acute pyrexia
- Tachycardia
- ± Hypotension
- Flushed
- Normal CVP.

± Predisposing cause

- Documented abscess
- Cholangitis
- Central venous catheter
- Wound infection
- Cellulitis
- Complication of GI surgery
- Post-urological procedure, with infected urine.

Management

- Blood cultures.

When appropriate

- Remove central line, send tip for culture
- Wound swab
- Urine for culture
- Drainage fluid culture
- Sputum culture.

Consult the patient's previous microbiology results because, if a septicaemic episode follows biliary or urinary tract surgery, the most likely agent of septicaemia will have been identified from previously performed bile/urine cultures.

- If the underlying cause is clear then treat accordingly.
- Septicaemia after abdominal surgery, with no obvious agent of infection, should be treated with broad-spectrum cephalosporin and metronidazole.
- Septicaemia after biliary surgery/procedures should be treated with piperacillin and gentamicin.

Postoperative chest infection
Pyrexia in the first/second postoperative day with minimal atelectasis and sputum retention should be treated with aggressive physiotherapy and mobilization and *not* antibiotics. Sputum should be sent for culture and sensitivity and antibiotics only commenced if the pyrexia persists and lung/CXR signs progress.

Antibiotic prophylaxis
Two, or at most three, doses covering a period of 8–16 h from the time of induction of anaesthesia for an operation are all that is required to reduce the virulence of an inoculum of organisms introduced during the procedure. It is not possible to 'protect' the patient against all pathogenic organisms he/she may encounter during the postoperative period.

Indications

Gastrointestinal surgery

- After the patient has been on H_2 antagonists – cephalosporin
- Hepatobiliary surgery
  - Cholecystectomy – cephalosporin
  - Bile duct procedure – cephalosporin
- Colorectal surgery – cephalosporin and metronidazole
- Appendicectomy – metronidazole.

Vascular surgery

- Flucloxacillin, ampicillin + cephalosporin for vascular reconstruction, particularly involving prosthetic grafts
- Benzylpenicillin, cephalosporin and metronidazole for leg amputation due to peripheral vascular disease.

Orthopaedic surgery

- Joint replacement – cephalosporin and/or gentamicin.

Other general points to remember when prescribing antibiotics

- Always take all of your culture samples before commencing antibiotics.

- Remember to ask patients about allergies, especially to penicillin. It is said that there is a 10% incidence of allergy to cephalosporins in patients who are allergic to penicillin.
- Be aware for signs of common antibiotic side-effects in your patients. These include candidiasis, for which it may be worth prescribing a prn dose of an antifungal cream, and diarrhoea in which pseudomembranous colitis should be considered.
- Warn women taking the OCP that antibiotics will reduce its efficacy and that they should use alternative methods of contraception.

ANALGESICS

Essentially, these are classified according to whether they are for:

- Minor pain (usually acute, short term)
- Moderate pain
- Severe pain (acute or chronic).

The management of severe pain, either postoperatively or in advanced malignancy, is best carried out in collaboration with your anaesthetic colleagues. Also, most hospitals have a specialist (usually an Anaesthetist) with an interest in the treatment of chronic pain. It may be appropriate to request their advice and assistance, since there are many nerve-blocking procedures that may help in achieving pain relief.

Minor pain

- *Aspirin* – oral 300–600 mg 4–6 hourly prn. Beware aspirin hypersensitivity and do not use in patients with a history of indigestion/peptic ulceration.
- *Paracetamol* – oral 0.5–1.0 g 6 hourly prn. Do *not* give in hepatic or renal impairment.
- *Ibuprofen* – oral 200–400 mg 6 hourly prn.

Moderate pain (3–14 days postoperatively)

Analgesics for moderate pain include the stronger NSAIDs (e.g. diclofenac 75 mg i.m. and ketorolac 30 mg i.m.) and the milder opioid drugs (e.g. codeine 30–60 mg orally and dihydrocodeine 25–50 mg i.v., 30–60 mg orally).

NSAIDs are particularly useful in treating musculoskeletal pain, e.g. following dental extraction, rib fractures, arthroscopy, dilatation and curettage.

Use compound preparations which combine simple analgesics (usually paracetamol) with small doses of opioids (e.g. codeine):

- *Co-dydramol* – oral 1–2 tablets 6 hourly prn
- *Co-proxamol* – oral 2 tablets 6–8 hourly prn.

Severe pain (immediate postoperative period and the management of chronic pain associated with malignancy) The strong analgesics comprise the opioid or morphine-like drugs

Morphine

- Oral preparations come as either Oramorph or sustained-release preparations such as MST and MXL. When prescribing morphine it is often best to begin by giving Oramorph on a prn basis for 24 h to assess the amount of analgesia required. Then convert this to a once or twice daily regular dose of a sustained-release preparation.
- i.m./subcutaneous – 10–20 mg 4 hourly prn (give with an antiemetic to reduce nausea).

Remember that exact dosage should be related to body weight and that the elderly are more sensitive to morphine. Also, in patients with poor renal function, the effects of a dose of morphine may be more prolonged and profound than expected, so care should be taken in titrating the dose for these patients.

Adverse effects

- Nausea (may be treated by conventional antiemetic drugs, e.g. metoclopramide and prochlorperazine or the strongest antiemeticum, which is haloperidol 1–2 mg)
- Vomiting
- Drowsiness
- Respiratory depression
- Constipation (in patients taking large doses, this is best treated by a combination of a bulking agent to soften the stool and a stimulant laxative to counteract the morphine-induced bowel stasis)
- Acute urinary retention
- Cutaneous itching, particularly of the nasal mucosa.

There are some myths to dispel about morphine:

- Addiction to morphine does not result from analgesic regimens.
- Despite reports of morphine causing spasm in the sphincter of Oddi, it is a perfectly satisfactory treatment for the pain of acute pancreatitis.

Also, morphine is extremely cheap (1 ampoule of 10 mg costs about 65 pence) and alternatives are more expensive.

Pethidine

Its effects are similar to those of morphine, except it has about one-tenth the potency (1 mg morphine = 10 mg pethidine).

Its duration of action is only 90–120 min and, if prescribed, this should be taken into account as it is not acceptable to prescribe pethidine '4–6 hourly as required'.

- Oral: 50–100 mg 3 hourly p.r.n.

- i.v./i.m.: 25–100 mg 3 hourly p.r.n. (may need to be given with an antiemetic because of nausea)

Diamorphine (heroin)

Its effects are identical to those of morphine, except that it is about twice as potent.

- i.m./i.v.: 5 mg 4–6 hourly prn.

Its use is reserved for the management of breakthrough pain in cancer and terminal illness.

Buprenorphine

This is less potent than morphine and its main advantage is that it can be given sublingually, which avoids hepatic first-pass metabolism.

Its duration of action is 6–8 h.

- Sublingual: 0.2–0.4 mg 4–6 hourly prn.

Adverse effects

- Nausea
- Drowsiness.

It is less prone to causing respiratory depression than morphine.

It is a partial agonist of opiate receptors and therefore should not be given in conjunction with conventional opiates.

Fentanyl

The patches are self-adhesive and transparent and applied to dry, non-irritated, non-irradiated skin. They provide a very stable therapeutic blood level and are wonderful in the treatment of chronic intractable pain due to cancer.

Adverse effects   See under morphine.

ANTICOAGULANTS

Anticoagulants are very commonly used in hospitals. Much of their use is in the treatment of pulmonary emboli and deep vein thrombosis and here we will concentrate on this; however, the guidelines can be applied to other clinical scenarios.

The potentially serious outcome associated with thrombo-embolic disease means that if there is reasonable clinical suspicion of a clot in either the veins or lungs then anticoagulation is almost unavoidable until the diagnosis can be confirmed.

If you are called to see a patient with a painful or swollen leg, or one who has suffered sudden pleuritic chest pain with or without haemoptysis, then you should assume that they have suffered a DVT or PE until proven one way or the other by radiological investigation. Confirmation of a DVT requires duplex Doppler studies of the leg or contrast venography.

Confirmation of a PE requires ECG changes (S1, Q3, T3 with right side strain), and or ventilation/perfusion isotope scan of the lungs, which demonstrates a ventilation perfusion mismatch (a region of lung field which is ventilated but not perfused). If these tests are unhelpful then the definitive investigation is pulmonary angiography.

The principles of treatment with anticoagulants are outlined below:

- Clinical decision made to anticoagulate.
- Send blood for baseline FBC, KCCT (APTT), INR, U&E.
- Arrange a confirmatory imaging test (within 24 h).
- For treatment of PE (and in some centres DVT) use intravenous unfractionated heparin (see heparin schedule below; Table 11.1).
- For treatment of DVT, subcutaneous low-molecular-weight heparin is now used in many centres. This has the advantage of requiring no monitoring except in patients with renal failure. Check local guidelines for dose; 200 units per kg in a single daily dose is often used (max. 18 000 units).
- Initiate warfarin once the diagnosis has been confirmed, and monitor INR daily as per schedule overleaf (Table 11.2). Heparin can be discontinued once the INR is in the appropriate therapeutic range.
- Arrange outpatient follow-up for warfarin therapy.
- If on heparin for more than 5 days, monitor platelet count daily.

Table 11.1
Heparin action with varying KCCT

KCCT ratio	Action
>7	Stop temporarily, wait 2 h and then recommence, reducing dose by 500 U/h
5.1–7.0	Reduced by 500 U/h
4.1–5.0	Reduce by 300 U/h
3.1–4.0	Reduce by 100 U/h
2.6–3.0	Reduce by 50 U/h
1.5–2.5	No change
1.2–1.4	Increase by 200 U/h
<1.2	Check the infusion pump is working. If it is, then increase the rate by 400 U/h. If this fails. seek haematological advice as the patient may well have a coagulation disorder

Table 11.2
Warfarin schedule

Day	INR (9 am)	Dose (mg) (6 pm)
1	<1.4	10.0
2	<1.8	10.0
	1.8	1.0
	>1.8	0.5
3	<2.0	10.0
	2.0–2.1	5.0
	2.2–2.3	4.5
	2.4–2.5	4.0
	2.6–2.7	3.5
	2.8–2.9	3.0
	3.0–3.1	2.5
	3.2–3.3	2.0
	3.4	1.5
	3.5	1.0
	3.6–4.0	0.5
	>4.0	0.0
4 (predicted maintenance dose)	<1.4	>8 (consult Haematology)
	1.4	8
	1.5	7.5
	1.6–1.7	7
	1.8	6.5
	1.9	6
	2.0–2.1	5.5
	2.2–2.3	5
	2.4–2.6	4.5
	2.7–3.0	4
	3.1–3.5	3.5
	3.6–4.0	3
	4.1–4.5	Miss out next day's dose and then give 2 mg
	>4.5	Miss out the next 2 days' doses and then given 1 mg

Heparin schedule (modified from Fennerty et al. *Br Med J* 1988; 297: 1285–8)

1. Loading dose: 5000 U over 5 min.
2. Commence infusion at 1400 U/h.
3. Check the KCCT after 6 h and adjust the rate of heparin infusion according to the ratio of the patient's KCCT compared with control values (Table 11.1).

Following any change in the rate of infusion, wait 10 h before the next KCCT ratio estimation. However, if the KCCT ratio is >5, then the next estimation should be made sooner, about 4 h later.

Anticoagulation treatment should continue for 1–3 months, and for at least 3 months in the case of a single recurrent thromboembolic episode. Patients under 45 years of age or with repeated thromboembolic episodes should be carefully investigated for underlying pathological processes, e.g. malignancy or thrombophilic disorders. They may require referral to a haematologist and possible life-long therapy.

Many hospitals now use APTT as a measure of heparin therapy; the schedule for dose alteration differs slightly so check local policy before initiating treatment.

GASTROINTESTINAL MEDICATION

ANTACIDS

The most commonly and widely used antacids are those that are based on salts of aluminium and magnesium. In addition, magnesium-containing compounds act as laxatives while aluminium-based antacids tend to cause constipation.

- *Aluminium hydroxide*: 1–2 tablets/pastilles 6 hourly prn
- *Magnesium trisilicate*: 10 ml suspension t.d.s. in water (may cause diarrhoea).

In addition to these simple preparations, further aluminium- and magnesium-based antacids are available, with both elements in combination with or without additional ingredients. Obviously these tend to be more expensive and of little proven benefit over the simple formulations.

DRUGS FOR PEPTIC ULCERS

Before prescribing blindly for indigestion, establish a diagnosis. Remember that the symptoms of peptic ulcer can mimic biliary colic, pancreatitis, angina, oesophagitis and other less common conditions. In addition, there is some benefit to be gained in prescribing these agents prophylactically in patients undergoing major surgery or having suffered severe trauma who have a history of peptic ulcer, bleeding diathesis, long-term NSAID administration or chronic steroid therapy.

H₂-receptor antagonists

These are probably best given in a course of 6–8 weeks, with ulcer healing then confirmed endoscopically. They have the advantage that they can be given both orally and parenterally.

- *Cimetidine* – oral: 400 mg b.d. or 800 mg nocte
  – i.v.: 200 mg 6 hourly
- *Ranitidine* – oral: 150 mg b.d.
  – i.v.: 50 mg 6–8 hourly
- *Famotidine* – oral: 40 mg nocte
- *Nizatidine* – oral: 150 mg b.d. or 300 mg nocte.

Sucralfate

A complex of aluminium hydroxide and sucrose sulphate, which is activated to bind to exudative proteinaceous surfaces at low pH (i.e. gastric acid).

- Oral: 2 g b.d. or 1 g 6 hourly.

Omeprazole

Omeprazole acts to inhibit gastric acid secretion by inhibiting the gastric parietal cell proton pump (H^+–K^+ adenosine triphosphatase pathway). Its major use is in the treatment of resistant ulcers, erosive oesophagitis and hypergastrinaemia due to Zollinger–Ellison syndrome.

Indications

- Peptic ulcer: 20 mg daily for 4–8 weeks
- Zollinger–Ellison syndrome: 60 mg daily
- Gastro-oesophageal reflux disease: 20 mg daily for 4–12 weeks, or longer in refractory oesophagitis.

Side-effects   Skin changes (rashes, urticaria, pruritus, alopecia), insomnia, diarrhoea, agitation.

Lansoprazole

Indications and side-effects
These are similar to those of omeprazole but side-effects vary per patient.

ANTIEMETICS

In surgical practice it is absolutely essential before antiemetics are prescribed for a patient who is vomiting, that a mechanical or septic cause for the vomiting is excluded. No amount of prescribing is going to divide an intestinal adhesion or drain a subphrenic abscess!

However, nausea and vomiting are frequent problems encountered by the House Surgeon. This is particularly the case in the postoperative period when recovering from general anaesthesia or receiving opioid analgesia and also when receiving cytotoxic chemotherapy.

- *Chlorpromazine* – oral: 10–25 mg 4–6 hourly prn
  – i.m.: 25 mg 4 hourly prn
  – p.r.: 100 mg 6–8 hourly prn
- *Domperidone* – oral: 10–20 mg 4–8 hourly prn
  – p.r.: 30–60 mg 8 hourly prn

- *Metoclopramide* – oral: 10 mg 8 hourly prn
  – i.m.: 10 mg 8 hourly prn.

Beware extrapyramidal side-effects, particularly oculogyric crisis.

- *Prochlorperazine* – oral: 5–10 mg 8 hourly prn
  – i.m.: 12.5 mg 6–8 hourly prn
- *Ondansetron* – oral: 8 mg 8 hourly.
  – i.m.: 8 mg 8 hourly.

This serotonin antagonist is a very expensive drug and should only be administered as an antiemetic during chemotherapy, particularly using cisplatinum compounds. Treatment should commence 2–3 h before chemotherapy, and continue for more than 2–3 days. It is also used as a one-dose shot in the immediate postoperative period after a laparoscopic Nissen fundoplication.

LAXATIVES

Bulk-forming agents

These agents act by increasing faecal mass, which in turn should stimulate peristalsis. By and large they are safe and non-toxic. Patients, particularly the elderly, often have little confidence in these agents because they do not produce an instant result. They should be warned that it will take several days before any appreciable improvement is noticed.

Bran and other sources of fibre are natural laxatives. Unfortunately, most hospital kitchens are loathe to allow anything that resembles healthy food leave their portals and head for the wards!

Commercially available bulk laxatives

- Ispaghula husk
  – Fybogel
  – Isogel
  – Metamucil
  – Regulan
- Methylcellulose
  – Celevac
- Sterculia
  – Normacol.

Reconstitute with water according to the manufacturer's guidelines and administer one to three times a day.

It is likely that your hospital pharmacy will have a bulk contract with the manufacturer of one of these agents, which will be the one you will end up using.

Contraindications

- Faecal impaction

- Intestinal obstruction
- Atonic bowel.

Stimulant laxatives

These agents act by irritating the bowel to stimulate intestinal motility. Because of this they may precipitate abdominal cramping pains.

- *Bisacodyl* (Dulco-lax)   – by mouth: 10 mg nocte
                              – by suppository: 10 mg mane
- *Cascara*   – by mouth: 20 mg nocte
- *Castor oil*   – by mouth: 10 ml nocte
- *Danthron* (co-danthrusate) – by mouth: 1–3 capsules nocte
  Beware reported carcinogenic risk
- *Docusate sodium* (Dioctyl)   – by mouth: up to 500 mg daily
- *Glycerol*   – by suppository: 1 prn
- *Senna* (Senokot)   – by mouth: 2–4 tablets nocte
- *Sodium picosulphate* (Picolax) – 1 sachet in water in the morning of the day before a colonic procedure, followed by a further sachet during the afternoon.

Contraindications

- Avoid in children
- Obstruction
- Prolonged overuse (misuse, particularly in the mentally unwell) can result in colonic atony and precipitate hypokalaemia.

Osmotic laxatives

These substances act by the osmotic retention of water in the stool, so loosening it and allowing freer passage.

- *Lactulose*   – by mouth: 15 ml
                                 elixir b.d.
- *Magnesium hydroxide* (liquid paraffin and magnesium hydroxide solution)   – by mouth: 5–20 ml prn
- *Magnesium sulphate* (Epsom salts) – by mouth: 5–10 mg in water, mane
                                 – by enema: 1 sachet prn
- *Phosphate enemas*   – by enema: 1 sachet prn.

Faecal softeners

These act both to soften and lubricate the stool.

- *Archis oil*   – by enema: 1 sachet prn
- *Liquid paraffin* – by mouth: 10–30 ml nocte.

TREATMENT OF DIARRHOEA

As in the treatment of vomiting and constipation, it is essential that before you blindly treat diarrhoea with any of the agents described below, you exclude a pathological or mechanical cause for the diarrhoea. In particular, in surgical patients look out for incomplete large bowel obstruction with faecal overflow, pseudomembranous colitis following antibiotic therapy, and a pelvic abscess following abdominal surgery.

Treatments for diarrhoea can be divided into two groups: drugs that reduce intestinal motility, and drugs that increase colonic adsorption.

Drugs reducing intestinal motility

- *Codeine phosphate* – oral: 10–60 mg 6 hourly prn
- *Loperamide* – oral: 4 mg followed by 2 mg after each loose stool (max. 16 mg daily).

Drugs increasing colonic adsorption

- *Kaolin* – oral: 10–30 ml of suspension 4–6 hourly prn.

BOWEL PREPARATION

It is necessary to cleanse and empty the colon of faecal residue before colonic surgery, colonoscopy and barium enema investigation. Traditional methods have involved admitting the patient days before surgery and keeping them on clear fluids with all sorts of dreadful purgatives. This was then changed to torturing the patient with a nasogastric tube down which warm normal saline was poured until the effluent ran out crystal clear at the other end. In most civilized units these methods have been superseded by the use of polyethylene glycol (sold under the proprietary names of Klean-Prep and Golytely).

Administration

1. Take at least 3–4 h after last solid food.
2. Reconstitute 1 sachet in 4 litres of water.
3. Take one tumblerful of this solution every 10–15 min until all 4 litres have been consumed or the resulting watery stools are free of solid matter.

The first bowel movement usually occurs after 1 h.

Adverse effects

- Nausea and bloating
- Abdominal cramps.

Contraindications to bowel prep

- Pregnancy
- Any evidence of intestinal obstruction
- Ulcerative colitis, especially toxic megacolon
- Stuporous or uncooperative patient, particularly when there may be loss of the gag reflex
- Gastric outflow obstruction
- Perforated bowel
- Peritonitis
- Body weight <20 kg.

12

Fluid and electrolyte balance and nutrition

FLUID AND ELECTROLYTE BALANCE

By many this is held to be mystical and regarded with great awe. This is absolute nonsense; you just need to follow a basic physiological principle: what comes out must be put back in.

What comes out?

Water

Put simply, in the normal physiological situation the losses are:

- Urine 1–2 litres/day
- Faeces 0.2 litres/day
- Insensitive losses 0.5 litres/day.

However, if your patient has diarrhoea, then faecal water losses will increase, but only by the amount you measure and so can be replaced. If your patient is febrile and/or the room is warm, then the insensitive losses will increase, upwards of 1 litre each day, but these insensitive losses cannot be measured easily.

Therefore, in a surgical patient who is given nil by mouth, but does not have any other abnormal fluid losses (nasogastric aspirate, fistula, diarrhoea, etc.), 3 litres of fluid volume each day will compensate for all normal water losses.

Electrolytes

From your point of view, the two most important are Na^+ and K^+. Losses of other electrolytes are also important and replacement of these is covered in total parenteral nutrition (see page 231). Daily Na^+ and K^+ losses in the normal physiological state are very similar at 80–90 mmol, the bulk of which is lost in urine, and some Na^+ in sweat. Therefore, this amount of both electrolytes should be added to your water replacement prescription.

The problem you are then faced with is making this fluid replacement isotonic with the extracellular fluid of the patient. The following solutions are known as the crystalloids and are isotonic:

- 5% dextrose
- Normal (0.9%) saline, containing 150 mmol of NaCl/litre
- Dextrose (4%) saline (0.18%), containing 30 mmol NaCl/litre
- Hartmann's solution
- Ringer's lactate solution.

Concentrate on the first three solutions. Consider the following 24 h fluid prescription:

- 1 litre normal saline with 20 mmol KCl over 8 h
- 1 litre 5% dextrose with 20 mmol KCl over 8 h
- 1 litre 5% dextrose with 20 mmol KCl over 8 h.

This will give the patient 3 litres of water (in an isotonic solution), 150 mmol of NaCl and 60 mmol of KCl. If the patient is not physiologically stressed and has normal renal and cardiac function, this prescription will be well tolerated and meet their normal fluid and electrolyte needs. Any excess water and sodium will be promptly excreted in the urine.

An alternative 24 h fluid prescription is:

- 1 litre dextrose saline with 20 mmol KCl over 8 h
- 1 litre dextrose saline with 20 mmol KCl over 8 h
- 1 litre dextrose saline with 20 mmol KCl over 8 h.

Again this will provide 3 litres of isotonic fluid and 60 mmol of K^+ during the 24 h period. However, Na^+ input will be reduced to 90 mmol (30 mmol in each litre of dextrose saline). This regimen is safer in a patient with cardiac impairment who is prone to fluid overload.

During the first 24 postoperative hours, there is a surge of adrenal steroids as a response to the stress and trauma of surgery. The consequence of this elevation in mineralocorticoids is Na^+ retention, at the expense of K^+ excretion. Therefore during this period, the safest fluid prescription for a patient with normal cardiac and renal function, and no other crystalloid losses is:

- 1 litre 5% dextrose with 20 mmol KCl over 8 h
- 1 litre 5% dextrose with 20 mmol KCl over 8 h
- 1 litre 5% dextrose with 20 mmol KCl over 8 h.

After the first 24 h revert to one of the other two regimens above, depending upon electrolyte balance and cardiac and renal function.

Excessive losses of water and electrolytes

Essentially these will occur in one of two situations:

- From the gut with nasogastric aspirates, fistula output and diarrhoea
- Polyuria.

However, the principles of management are the same. Measure the volume of the abnormal loss of fluid and incorporate this volume with the standard 3 litres a day lost. Therefore, if the loss is in nasogastric aspirate or fistula output, add it to the standard 3 litres out each day. If the loss is due to polyuria, incorporate it into the formula previously described, replacing the normal urinary volume loss of 2 litres/day with the patient's measured daily output.

In addition, measure the electrolyte concentration of the losses and the ABG concentrations. The Na^+ concentration of GI secretions is to all intents and purposes the same as serum. However, K^+ concentrations vary, being the same as serum in most GI secretions, but as high as 8 mmol/l in gastric secretions. Measure the Na^+ and K^+ concentrations in the urine and the aspirate/fistula output and calculate the electrolyte replacement requirements as follows:

- Total urinary Na^+ and K^+ losses
- Total aspirate/fistula Na^+ and K^+ losses.

Having measured the total water (volume) and electrolytes lost, prescribe the fluid replacements required. In practice, this usually amounts over a 24 h period to:

- 1 litre dextrose saline with 20 mmol KCl
- 1 litre dextrose saline with 20 mmol KCl
- 1 litre dextrose saline with 20 mmol KCl
- Additional replacement using normal saline with appropriate addition of KCl.

In addition, if the excessive losses are from the upper gut, you will have to compensate for the electrolyte losses due to acid–base imbalance (see page 227). Excessive nasogastric aspirate/vomiting will produce a loss of H^+ with a resulting metabolic alkalosis. To compensate, the distal renal tubules will try to conserve H^+ by actively exchanging them for K^+. So, in addition to the metabolic alkalosis, there will be an associated hypokalaemia, which will require compensation. Excessive losses from a pancreatic fistula will include large amounts of bicarbonate, which occasionally may result in a metabolic acidosis and require bicarbonate replacement.

Management of Na^+ and K^+ imbalance

Hyponatraemia
In a surgical patient this is usually due to water overload. Avoid using saline. Instead, fluid restrict your patient to 1–2 litres/day and diurese for 48 h using frusemide 40 mg b.d. Monitor the electrolytes twice daily during this time.

Hypernatraemia
In a surgical patient this is uncommon. The two situations in which it will arise are dehydration and during the immediate postoperative period when inappropriate mineralocorticoid secretion will cause Na^+ retention. Dehydration (clinically dry, low CVP, oliguria) will need water replacement, whereas post-operative hypernatraemia in the presence of normal hydration is managed by Na^+ restriction (see above).

Hypokalaemia
In a surgical patient this is usually due to inadequate K^+ replacement, particularly when a patient is receiving K^+-depleting diuretics. The other 'surgical' situation in which hypokalaemia is part of the clinical picture is pyloric stenosis. As a consequence of prolonged loss of H^+ from the stomach (resulting in a metabolic alkalosis), there is renal compensation by exchanging H^+ for K^+ in the distal renal tubule. Hypo-kalaemia is associated with T-wave flattening on the ECG. The

onset may be insidious and may be the cause of a prolonged postoperative ileus. The treatment is K^+ replacement.

Hyperkalaemia

A K^+ of >7 mmol/l is an emergency. In surgical patients it is usually associated with acute renal failure. The other cause of hyperkalaemia seen in surgical patients is massive tissue destruction (crush or burn injuries) when K^+ leaks out of the traumatized tissues. Beware the diagnosis of hyperkalaemia being made on a haemolysed blood sample. Hyperkalaemia is associated with T-wave elevation on the ECG. Start treatment by giving 10% calcium gluconate (20 ml) over 5 min to protect the heart cells, then give 100 ml of 8.4% sodium bicarbonate to correct any acidosis. Fifteen units of soluble insulin with 50 g glucose is given as a rapid infusion to push the K^+ back into the cells. Repeated calcium resonium enemas (20 g t.d.s.) are given to remove K^+ from the body. Arrange dialysis if K^+ is persistently high. Most important is that the cause of the hyperkalaemia should be addressed as soon as possible.

Acid–base imbalance

The common causes of acid – base imbalance in a surgical patient are (Table 12.1):

- *Respiratory acidosis*:
  - Atelectasis and sputum retention (treat with physiotherapy)
  - Massive pulmonary embolism
- *Respiratory alkalosis*:
  - Hyperventilation due to anxiety
- *Metabolic acidosis*:
  - Septic, hypovolaemic or cardiogenic shock
- *Metabolic alkalosis*:
  - Gastric outflow obstruction, pyloric stenosis.

To determine the nature of the imbalance, measure the pH and the arterial CO_2 ($PaCO_2$) concentration.

Table 12.1 Acid – base imbalance		
Imbalance	pH	$PaCO_2$
Respiratory acidosis	↓	↑
Respiratory alkalosis	↑	↓
Metabolic acidosis	↓	↓*
Metabolic alkalosis	↑	↑*
Due to attempted respiratory compensation.		

Blood and colloid replacement

The circulatory volume is about 4 litres, of which 35–40% is made up of cells (99% red blood cells) and the remainder is plasma (water, proteins: albumin, clotting factors, globulins). In addition the water of this extracellular component may communicate with the other body water compartments: the extracellular and intracellular fluids, which constitute 10 and 25 litres respectively in a 70 kg man.

In the situation of hypovolaemic shock (i.e. the loss of circulating blood volume) the purpose of therapy is to restore the circulating volume using colloids. This may sound obvious but it is surprising how many people qualify in medicine and do not know the difference between crystalloids and colloids:

- *Crystalloids* are solutions of salts and/or sugars in water, which equilibrate with the total extracellular body water.
- *Colloids* contain macromolecules in water which equilibrate only in the intravascular compartment, e.g. albumin solution.

If the problem is one of bleeding, then the best replacement fluid is blood, ideally cross-matched to the patient's own blood. Transfusion for hypovolaemic shock must be carried out against the physiological measurements of the patient's arterial blood pressure, CVP urine output and haematocrit (see cardio-pulmonary resuscitation, pages 88, 94).

> **Remember**
>
> In cases of torrential haemorrhage and profound hypo-volaemic shock, the universal blood donor is O negative and the universal recipient is AB positive.

If the problem is one of volume loss without actual bleeding, as manifested by oliguria and a low CVP (fluid sequestration following burns, acute pancreatitis or any other cause of a large raw surface), then the treatment is colloid replacement:

- Low CVP, normal albumin, normal clotting: give an artificial colloid, e.g. Gelofusine or Haemaccel, as a fluid challenge.
- Low CVP, low albumin, normal clotting: give 4.5% albumin solution ('plasma'). You will probably have to discuss the use of this expensive item with the Haematology Department.
- Abnormal clotting with an elevated INR: give fresh frozen plasma, 6–10 U and measure the INR. In addition give 20 mg of vitamin K.
- Abnormal clotting due to low platelets (<80 000/ml^3) and a prolonged bleeding time: give 6–10 U of platelets.

Poor urine output (see also page 91)

This is a frequent problem on the surgical ward, particularly in the postoperative period. Postoperative oliguria (<500 ml urine/24 h, <30 ml urine/h) is abnormal and unacceptable. Anuria in a surgical patient is an emergency!

There are three causes of acute renal failure in a surgical patient:

- *Pre-renal* due to poor cardiac output, i.e. shock, which may be cardiogenic, hypovolaemic or septic.
- *Renal* as a consequence of renal ischaemia, particularly in diabetics and arteriopaths.
- *Post-renal* due to obstruction of the urinary tract. The two most common causes of this in a surgical patient are acute retention due to prostatism and a blocked catheter.

The management of poor renal output in a surgical patient is as follows:

1. Check the blood pressure; if normotensive, catheterize.
2. If there is already a catheter in place, then flush it to ensure that it is not blocked.
3. If the catheter is patent and/or the patient is hypotensive, place a central venous catheter and measure the CVP (see page 179). Correct the hypovolaemia to restore the CVP to +10 cmH$_2$O, initially with colloid.
4. Review the urine output over the next 15 min.
5. If still no response, then start a renal dose of dopamine (2–5 µg/kg/min) at the lowest dose.

If none of these manoeuvres works, your patient has acute renal failure. This is a medical emergency and you should consult the Renal Physicians immediately. *On no account give frusemide and hope.*

NUTRITIONAL SUPPORT

Indications

- *Preoperatively* in malnourished patients so that they regain weight lost due to chronic illness and are in the best condition for major surgery.
- *Postoperatively* for malnourished patients to allow them to recover from major surgery and to encourage wound healing.
- *Long-term* in cases where nutrition is inadequate for any reason.

Nutritional support may be enteral or parenteral.

Enteral nutritional support

1. *Oral*
   – A diet with a high concentration of whatever is required (e.g. protein, high calorie).

2. *Narrow-bore nasogastric tube*
   – If oral supplementation is inadequate
   – 1 mm internal diameter, polyethylene or silastic tubes
     are soft and require a guide wire for insertion and
     changing (every few months)
   – To give supplemental feeding gradually over long
     periods, such as at night.
3. *Gastrostomy*
   – For patients with abnormality of the mouth, pharynx or
     oesophagus. This can be congenital or acquired.
   – A percutaneous endoscopic gastrostomy (PEG) is given
     under LA if the stomach is accessible with endoscopy.
4. *Jejunostomy*
   – Needs a GA but preferably done at initial operation
   – A 1 mm internal catheter is inserted into the jejunum via
     a submucosal tunnel
   – In conditions where a nasogastric tube cannot be used
     (fistula, obstruction or recently made anastomosis of the
     upper GI tract) and delayed oral feeding is anticipated
     or where long-term enteral nutrition is required
   – Possible complications: leakage, adhesions and volvulus
     of the bowel.

In patients with an intact and functioning gut who need
nutritional support, enteral nutrition is preferable to parenteral
nutrition because it is:

● Cheaper (minimal medical staff involved)
● Safe and simple
● Maintains integrity of gut mucosa and reduces the risk of
  bacterial translocation.

Initial feeding is best administered at quarter strength, rapidly
building up to full strength using any of the commercially
available feed mixtures. Rate of administration is best regulated
using an infusion control pump.

One complication is diarrhoea, especially if the patient has
not been enterally fed for some time, with resulting jejunal
mucosal atrophy. If it occurs then reduce the strength of the
feed and build up again slowly.

Parenteral feeding (intravenous nutrition)

1. *Peripheral feeding*
   – Only for the short term (expected to take adequate oral
     food in about 7 days)
   – Can only involve types of feed (with lower osmolarity)
     that do not cause thrombophlebitis
   – Thrombophlebitis can be minimized by diluting the
     solution with fluid, or by the addition of heparin or
     hydrocortisone (5 mg) to each litre of solution.
2. *Central venous feeding*
   – This may be a simple percutaneous line (for short-term

use) or an indwelling subcutaneous line (Hickman or Nutricath), placed operatively into the cephalic, internal or external jugular or subclavian vein

– Subcutaneous ports are available for long-term parenteral support (for conditions such as severe Crohn's disease, small bowel malnutrition or short bowel syndrome). The patients are taught how to introduce the food with a sterile set into the central venous circulation.

Long-term central lines require operative conditions to be placed and are not devoid of problems:

- Insertion of the cannula can cause air embolism, pneumothorax or thrombosis of major veins.
- Line sepsis as a result of prolonged access to the circulation via the catheter. (Resist the tendency to remove the line in a pyrexial patient unless cultures of blood withdrawn through the line are positive, although the degree of sepsis may be such that earlier removal of the line is mandatory.)
- A period of 48 h is mandatory between the removal of an infected line and the placement of a new one to avoid metastatic infection.

It is often worth deferring the placement of an indwelling line by using a simple percutaneous line until it is clear that long-term feeding is going to be required.

TOTAL PARENTERAL NUTRITION

Total parenteral nutrition has revolutionized clinical medicine over the last decade. With specific regard to routine surgical practice it is now feasible to feed malnourished and starving patients before and after major surgery during which the GI tract is out of action for prolonged periods.

The decision to commence TPN should be taken at a senior level and should be made at the very latest on the morning ward round of the day it is to commence. Subsequent decisions to continue feeding and review nutritional requirements must be made before lunchtime in order to deliver the necessary prescription to the Pharmacy. Most district hospital pharmacies now provide large (up to 3 litre) bags of ready made up TPN (either prepared in their own laboratory or purchased complete). Most pharmacies in the UK use brand regimen products with added supplements from other companies. The advice below is based on these regimens and should be altered after consultation with your own pharmacy to adapt to local conditions (see Table 12.2).

The following are also found in all regimens (Table 12.3):

- *Trace elements*: Addamel given daily in all regimens
- *Vitamins*: Solivito and Vitlipid 1 vial daily (Monday to Friday only as not stable enough to last the weekend).

Table 12.2
Parenteral nutrition regimens

Clinical requirements	Kabivitrum regimen	Volume (litres)	Calories (kcal)	Nitrogen (g)	Na^{++} (mmol)	K^{++} (mmol)	Ca^{2+} (mmol)
Normal	Kabi 1	2.25	2100	9	65 200	55 150	7.5
Modestly increased	Kabi 3	3	2400	14	98 240	93 180	8.8
Fluid and sodium restricted	Kabi 2a	2	2000	9	15 160	15 120	5.0

*The first figure refers to the normal electrolyte content. The figure underneath is the maximum electrolyte content after further addition (on request).

Table 12.3
Trace elements and vitamins

Addamel		Solivito		Vitlipid	
Ca^{2+}	5.0 mmol	B1		1.2 mg	Retinol (A) 750 µg (2500 U)
Mg^{2+}	1.5 mmol	B2		1.8 mg	
Fe^{3+}	50.0 µmol				
Zn^{2+}	20.0 µmol	Nicotinamide		10.0 mg	Calciferol (D2) 3 µg (120 U)
Mn^{2+}	40.0 µmol	B6		2.0 mg	
Cu^+	5.0 µmol	Pantothenic acid		10.0 mg	Phytomenadione 150 µg
F^-	50.0 µmol	Biotin		0.3 mg	
I^-	1.0 µmol	Folic acid		0.2 µg	Also contains fractionated soya
Cl^-	13.3 mmol	B12		2.0 µg	bean oil (1 g), egg
		C		30 mg	phospholipids (120 mg)
					and glycerol (225 mg)

Multibionta

If higher initial vitamin treatment is indicated or routinely if feeding continues for more than 2 weeks, Multibionta is given on Tuesday and Thursday instead of Solivito. It contains the following vitamins:

A 10 000 U
B1 50 mg
B2 10 mg
B6 15 mg
Nicotinamide 100 mg
Pantothenyl alcohol 25 mg
C 500 mg
E 5 mg

Not included in TPN but recommended to be given independently are:

- Folic acid injection 15 mg i.m. once a week
- Hydroxycobalamin injection 1 mg i.m. every 2 weeks
- Iron (as iron dextran: imferon) by i.m. injection as appropriate.

Catheter insertion

It is possible to administer TPN to patients via the peripheral veins. However, this requires meticulous care with regard to cannulae, which must be either replaced daily, or kept open with the regular application of GTN skin patches distal to the cannula (to keep the vein dilated). It is usually logistically simpler and kinder to the patient to use a central venous catheter for TPN, but this again requires meticulous care with regard to insertion and also to avoid air embolism.

Long catheters placed centrally via the antecubital vein at the elbow may allow feeding for several days and are relatively safe. However, they are difficult to manage from the nursing point of view.

Prolonged TPN is best given via a tunnelled subclavicular catheter, which can now be performed using percutaneous puncture for all steps. While direct percutaneous puncture can be performed in the ICU or ward, it is preferable that a TPN catheter be placed in the operating theatre (see insertion of central venous catheter, page 179).

For patients with complex problems, such as those in whom TPN is to be administered simultaneously with other i.v. drugs and/or central venous pressure measurements, then double and triple lumen catheters are available.

Biochemical monitoring

It is usual to inform the Biochemistry Laboratory that a patient is about to start TPN; in some hospitals this is mandatory. All subsequent biochemistry request forms should state that the patient is on TPN, and samples should reach the laboratory first thing in the morning to ensure inclusion on that morning's routine run. Twenty-four hour urine collections should commence at 8.00 am. Electrolyte results should be available by lunchtime so that alterations can be made to the next 24 h prescription.

All patients receiving TPN should be carefully monitored and their progress documented. The best way to do this is to construct a flow chart which includes all haematological and biochemical values in addition to the patient's weight and fluid/nitrogen balance.

- Before starting:
  - Venous blood
    - U & E
    - Creatinine
    - Urate
    - Glucose
    - Calcium
    - Phosphate
    - LFTs, particularly albumin and bilirubin
    - Magnesium
  - Arterial blood
    - Gas and acid – base status as clinically indicated
  - Urine
    - U & E (urinary urea being used as a major guide to nitrogen balance)
- Until fluid and nitrogen balance obtained:
  - 6 hourly BM Stix to measure blood sugar
  - Daily
    - Serum U & E
    - Urine: 24 h collection for U & E; ward testing (ketones, protein glucose, pH)
  - × 3 weekly
    - Calcium
    - Phosphate
    - LFTs
  - Daily weight charted
- Once fluid and nitrogen balance obtained:
  - Twice weekly
    - U & E
    - Calcium
    - Phosphate
    - LFTs
- Weekly
  - Magnesium
- If indicated:
  - Iron
  - Total iron-binding capacity
  - Zinc.

Sepsis

Sepsis is suspected if there is unexplained pyrexia or unexpected glucose intolerance.

You should arrange for culture of:

- Blood from a peripheral vein
- Draw-back blood from the feeding line
- Wound swab
- Swab from the catheter insertion site
- MSU/CSU
- Sputum
- A sample of TPN from the TPN bag

and change the TPN bag and giving set.

If there is an obvious cause of sepsis, treat with an appropriate antibiotic; if still pyrexial after 24 h, consider removal of the feeding line. If apyrexial after 24 h, continue antibiotics and leave the feeding line in place.

If there is no obvious source of sepsis, consider removing the feeding line. If apyrexial after 24 h, insert a new feeding line; however, if pyrexial, commence antibiotics. If the line is removed, send the tip to Microbiology for culture and sensitivity.

SECTION 4

Surviving as a junior doctor

13

Professional relationships

WORKING IN A TEAM

For many of you this will be your first permanent job. Whether you are working for 3, 6 or 12 months in the same hospital you need to develop a good relationship with your colleagues.

General points

It is no longer the case that doctors run hospitals; like it or not, you are now a small part of a huge healthcare team. Each person has their own job and you must respect that their priorities may be different to yours. As a rule, if you are polite and explain your request fully, people will respond in the way you want. Make sure that before you contact anyone to request their help you have all the available information; it's no good requesting an urgent CT scan because 'my consultant asked for it'. If they are adamant that your request is not appropriate, either ask them to contact your immediate senior or, if you are certain of your position, inform them that you will be documenting their name and decision in the notes. It's amazing how often the blood test gets done when the technician realises that he or she will be held legally responsible for the clinical consequences.

Nurses

Worthy of special mention, nursing staff can be your greatest ally or worst enemy. Even the most junior Staff Nurse will have spent 2 or 3 years working on a ward, and although they may not have the theoretical knowledge, they will have far more practical experience than you. Nurses are not there as your assistant, they have their own specific role in the care of the patient; however, they are normally happy to help you out, either with practical advice or when performing a procedure, *if you are nice to them!*

If you are asked to do something by a nurse that you feel is inappropriate, don't just refuse and storm off, grumbling about how awful all nurse are! It is unlikely that she has asked you to do it just to wind you up, so ask her why she wants it done and then explain your reason for not doing it. If she is insistent, then speak to the Ward Sister about it. If it is in the middle of the night it might be better to spend 5 min doing the job and have a quiet word with the Ward Sister the next day, rather than refuse and spend the next hour lying awake all worked up (the nurse won't be!!).

TALKING TO PATIENTS AND THEIR RELATIVES

Talking to patients and their relatives is an important part of the House Surgeon's job. The way in which the entire surgical team is regarded by the patient may depend on this. Although it is frequently desirable that someone more senior should discuss particular points, such as a serious diagnosis (e.g. cancer) or the implications of a major operation, it is often the case that the House Surgeon is the only person available when the relatives are around. The following points may help to make this job easier.

Patients

You must be honest with patients, but you need not be brutally honest. It is often fairly easy to discover how much a patient wishes to know about their condition by asking questions such as, 'Is there anything more that you want to know?' or, 'Would you like to ask me any questions?'. The patient may then give a firmly negative response, or they may ask frank questions. In either case you need to know how to handle these.

The patient who gives a negative response when invited to discuss their diagnosis or prognosis has very often decided that they have a terminal illness. If this is indeed the case there may be little to be gained from labouring the point, although the patient may assume the worst so that encouragement or support may still be useful.

The patient who wants a frank discussion deserves exactly that. Do not attempt to fob patients off with generalizations. If the prognosis for a particular condition is known, and the patient wishes to know it, they must be told. This, of course, assumes that you know the correct answer. If you are unsure about details of prognosis, say so. It is much better to say, 'I'm not sure about that, but I will find the answer out and come back later to discuss it', than to give a wrong answer. It is also very important to remember that prognostic figures are statistical estimates for a whole group of patients. It is not usually possible to give a prognostic assessment which is accurate, even when life expectancy is very short, so try to avoid being too specific.

Relatives

Most of the points made about talking to patients can be applied to talking to relatives. There are, however, a few important points. Relatives have no statutory right to confidential information about patients. Although, in practice, you will often speak quite openly to relatives, your first duty is to the patient. If the patient asks you not to reveal a diagnosis to a relative you are bound to confidentiality. Relatives who ask you not to discuss diagnosis or prognosis with patients need to be dealt with sympathetically, but firmly. A response such as, 'Of course I won't force anything down his throat but if he asks me a direct question then I'll answer', usually works. Although acceptance of an adverse diagnosis and a poor prognosis is painful, once done it allows honest discussion to take place. A family situation where everyone has guessed the diagnosis but no-one admits it prevents admission of symptoms (which are usually controllable) and emotional support.

> ### Remember
>
> The key points when talking to either patients or relatives are *honesty*, *mutual trust* and *factual accuracy* wherever the facts are available to make this possible.

THE LAW

The police

You may come across the police in a number of circumstances. The most common situation by far is in A & E, and this is the place where most mistakes are made in general and in dealing with the police in particular. Remember the following:

- Your responsibility to a patient's confidentiality remains the same whether the person asking you about that patient is a civilian or a police officer.
- If you believe that withholding information about a patient's possible criminal activities may place in danger the life of another person, then you are at liberty to divulge what information you believe is necessary.
- You may be required to give the name (and name only) of any person involved in a road traffic accident. Do not, however, be bullied by the police into giving confidential information in other non-violent crimes. There are approved channels to obtain such information if it is required and you should simply state that you are too junior to divulge it and that they should refer to your superior.
- You are not at liberty to carry out tests such as blood alcohol levels (or physical examination for the ingestion of drugs) without the consent of the patient, since this may constitute an assault unless the test is required to diagnose the cause of drowsiness or unconciousness. In any case the rules of confidentiality should be applied.

> ### Remember
>
> Most of the police you will encounter in A & E are junior and have a scanty knowledge of the law as applied to confidentiality. They are not used to being told that information is not available to them. You can deal with this in two opposing ways: appear to know more than they do and try to dominate the situation, or appear to know nothing and refer the matter upwards.

- You may be asked to give an account of a patient's injuries and what you think may have caused them. If you are not trained in forensic science you would be unwise to give any details of the likely causes of an injury except in the most vague form.

Legal reports

You may be asked from time to time to supply reports for the police. There is usually a fee attached to this so don't forget to declare it on your tax form. If you are inexperienced at filling in forms it is wise to get a more experienced doctor to look over its content before you return it. If it contains any information that is from the patient's notes, and is therefore confidential, it cannot be released without an appropriate subpoena or a written letter of consent from the patient or their solicitor. If you err in this way you may be in breach of confidentiality. Lawyers occasionally will send you a charming letter asking for confidential information, claiming to act on behalf of the client. *Do not release any information without the written permission of that client.* The lawyer may turn out to be acting for the other side.

Appearing in court

If you are called to court, this will be either to give evidence about a patient, usually in relation to an accident or an assault, or to defend yourself, if a patient has brought a complaint. In the latter case you should be represented in court. *In either case, you would be wise to scrutinize the notes in detail and to read around the subject.* Lawyers can be extremely precise in their questioning and if you are unprepared you can be made to look a fool. Stick absolutely to what you know and don't be drawn into conversations beyond your expertise; you will be there as a witness to fact and not opinion. If what they need is an expert opinion, they can employ one. If you start to give medical opinions they will destroy you. Humble factuality is by far the best bet. Always seek advice early either from the professional organizations, such as the MDU, or from health authority lawyers.

THE MEDIA

From time to time you may find yourself the subject of media attention. This may be because of a situation you have become involved in (such as a major accident) or you may have your opinion sought because of your position or your post. Whatever the circumstance there are a number of points to bear in mind:

- You are an ambassador for your profession – speak sensibly and seriously.
- You are an ambassador for your institution – don't denigrate your hospital.

Reporters of all kinds may be happy to encourage an indiscreet remark. Reporters from some major newspapers appear particularly unscrupulous in their use of sources of information. Ask yourself:

- Would comment on a particular issue infringe patient confidentiality?
- Are you qualified to comment; should any comment instead come from a superior?
- Is the comment appropriate for a doctor; should it come from an administrator?
- Are you free to comment; do you have a contractual obligation to stay silent?

> **Remember**
>
> You may have considerable opportunity to regret a few words spoken in haste. If in doubt, keep quiet.

TAX AND THE HOUSE OFFICER

This can appear misleadingly complicated. Your earnings are taxed at source, so provided you have no additional earnings and wish to make no additional allowance claims, all you need do is forward your P60 each year and the Inland Revenue will do the rest. However, your situation is unlikely to be as straightforward as this because you are almost certain to make some small additional earnings and you will be entitled to make some claims against tax.

Tax-deductible professional expenses

- Membership to professional bodies, e.g. the GMC, BMA or MDU
- Membership to medical societies, e.g. the Surgical Research Society
- Essential medical equipment (ophthalmoscope, stethoscope), although tax officers can be a little more sticky about this and sometimes claiming for this is not worth the trouble.

Additional earnings

You must make a note of incidental earnings and declare these. The tax office has a habit of retrospectively billing you for what it thinks you may have earned, just because it found one or two items which you omitted to declare in your younger and more innocent days. The additional earnings that are particularly easy to trace are:

- Cremation forms (ash cash)

- Police reports
- Insurance reports
- Assistant fees for private operations
- Gifts for looking after private patients and gifts from patients in cash or kind. (The tax office is unlikely to require you to record every chocolate that you eat at the nurses station, but anything more substantial may be taxable.)

Generally speaking, a good accountant can be found who will charge you very little and may help both to reduce your tax bill and the burden of administration in filling in your tax return. If you don't receive a tax form, this is because the Inland Revenue assumes you have no other earnings. You should write and ask for one because you can at least make claims for your professional expenses. If you have any questions and don't have an accountant, the tax office is, surprisingly, often very helpful in sorting things out. If you are the unfortunate recipient of a large bill for income that you didn't earn, but which the tax office thinks you may have, then you are entitled to insist that it identifies the precise earnings. The employment of an accountant as an emergency measure may be deemed wise at this stage. Otherwise plead ignorance, innocence and ask for help from the tax office, who will have to tell you in the end what it thinks you have earned and why.

PERSONAL HEALTH ('CAN I COPE?')

You may have no problem coping – nevertheless read on! The advice below is written for three groups of people. The first, and most obvious group, is 'the stressed'. The trouble is that stressed people don't have much time to read or may not know where to look for help, which is half their problem. The second group of people is 'the bystanders', who are not themselves particularly prone to stress but amongst those who are. If you are in this group, read what follows so that you can recognize the symptoms of stress and help your colleagues if need be. The third group is 'the stressors', the people who, accidentally or deliberately, stress others. If those around you (particularly those junior to you) start to manifest symptoms of stress, you should, if you've an ounce of decency in you, recognize this and change your behaviour.

Stress is a major topic of conversation amongst junior hospital staff and the sporadic suicide reflects the tip of an iceberg of overwork, loneliness and despair. Whilst some of the moves to reduce doctors' hours may improve this situation, it is not overwork alone that leads to problems. Problems are many and multifactorial and rarely manifest in a straightforward way, but as various symptoms of failure to cope.

The problems

Loneliness

This is not the same as being alone. In this context loneliness means isolation from those with whom problems can be aired, shared, empathized with and talked through. One of the most reassuring discoveries when everything seems to be getting out of hand is that your peers feel the same way. *You're normal – it's not just you.* Isolated from this reassurance and the normalizing influence of others, even small problems grow into huge ones.

Tiredness/physical illness

Tiredness is likely to continue to be the lot of the junior doctor for the foreseeable future. Even with the introduction of less onerous rotas you will still have to work substantially harder than most people outside medicine and the shift-type systems will mean that you are working harder when you are on-call. Illness multiplies these problems and tiredness and illness have a more than additive effect.

Too much work

There may be times when you feel you have too much work to do or you may feel this way all the time. The problem may be overload or it may be that organization and prioritization are at fault.

Too much responsibility

There are two problems here. First, you may be asked to make decisions and implement actions for which you have not yet acquired the necessary experience. You are being given too much responsibility. Second, you may be asked to get things done but do not have the authority to make them happen. For instance, you may be told to get a test done today, but you haven't the authority to demand that the appropriate department does it for you. Either of these situations can be stressful, particularly responsibility without authority.

Difficult working relations

This is usually at the heart of many other problems. The reason that you have too much work or responsibility is that someone else up the line is dumping it on you. There are people who feel it is their duty to make the House Officer scuttle around the whole time; others remember having a hard time and can't wait to get their own back by making someone else's life more difficult. Sometimes the problem is just that people are difficult to talk to so that easy problems can't be aired and solved. Like so many other things it seems that the people who most need the support of others are the least able to get it. This insecurity can be manifest as defensiveness or even aggression, thus worsening the situation.

The symptoms

Drink

Drinking has been part of the medical student scene for centuries and seems unlikely to disappear. Alcohol, taken in moderation, is no bad thing, but stress can lead to drinking getting out of control. The signs are well known: gradually increasing consumption, inability to get to work on time, particularly after a weekend off, smelling of alcohol in the morning and drinking on-call.

Absenteeism

One manifestation of an unhappy work situation is absenteeism. This is particularly common amongst nursing staff. In a way it can be reassuring: someone with the confidence to take time off, under whatever pretext, is usually sufficiently in charge of themselves to recognize problems and see a solution, even if it is temporary and only partially satisfactory. If you see this in your colleagues or juniors suspect problems rather than idleness (although it may be the latter).

Anger and irritability

Happy people are easy to get on with. Colleagues who are consistently cross or irritable are probably in trouble emotionally. This may not be much help (you are not recommended to invite your Consultant who has the personality of an enraged bull to discuss his problems with you), but at least you may be able to keep things in perspective. If you find yourself getting more and more irritable, stress is likely to be the cause.

Burnout

This phenomenon appears to occur when the ability to cope with stress is exceeded. Symptoms before final crisis include irritability, anxiety, frustration, anger, resentment, guilt, apathy and cynicism. This may be associated with coffee all day to keep going and alcohol at night to get to sleep. There may be associated physical illness such as ulcers. The result is a complete inability to cope with anything. This may manifest as a form of absenteeism or a failure to do any work at all. Prolonged rest seems to be the only cure. The problem can recur.

So far so bad, now what?

Seen from the outside nothing that you are going through is really that bad. After all you are healthy (probably), adequately fed and housed (hopefully), and in work (definitely), but perspective is lost. Real problems are left unsolved and small problems grow into big ones. What should you do?

Loneliness

Early in your appointment make a point of introducing yourself to nursing and other staff around the hospital with whom you will be working, so that they know you by name. This is particularly important if you are moving to a new hospital where you know few of the other staff. Similarly, it is worth meeting other junior staff where you can, and making a point of going to the doctors' mess for meals, rather than just eating sandwiches, so that generally you get to know people. Joining local clubs or other activities will help to build a network of contacts outside the working environment, which can help greatly in maintaining your equilibrium – meet 'normal' people in 'normal' jobs. Time spent socializing, both at work and in your spare time, can seem to be wasted. It isn't, you need it, so fit it in somehow. If things are getting out of hand, talk to other members of staff, particularly those who seem sympathetic. Which particular members these will be, you will have to decide for yourself. There is almost always a hospital chaplain and, whatever your religion or faith may be, they have long experience of giving confidential advice.

Tiredness/physical illness

If you are tired, go to bed and sleep. There is a strong temptation when newly qualified to try to do everything you did as a student as well as being a House Officer, particularly since you may have rather more money to spend now. This is rarely realistic and it is better to save your energy and money for when you are fresh than to exhaust yourself after a busy night on-call.

If you are unwell, resist the pressure to stay at work whatever happens. There are people who feel that you either come to hospital as a doctor or as a patient! This is ridiculous. If you are ill you will get better much faster, and be more efficient overall, if you take off sufficient time to recuperate. Don't overdo this though or your return to work may be stormy, and try not to get spotted shopping or at the cinema whilst off sick.

Too much work

If you cannot cope with all the work you have to do then do the most important jobs first. Make a list of the priorities and stick to them. It is easy to get carried away spending time on trivial tasks. Try to delegate wherever possible; filing can be done by nurses at night if they are not busy, but it all depends on how nicely you ask. If you still can't manage, tell your superiors that you can't do everything and ask what can be left out? Don't whinge to the Consultant about your colleagues as this will do nothing for professional relationships.

Too much responsibility

If you are asked to take decisions or perform procedures for which you have insufficient expertise, say so. The person delegating is responsible for your mistakes. If you have been given responsibilities but haven't the authority to make things happen, say so. The person delegating can then intervene. Don't let anyone tell you that you are at fault. You are not.

Difficult working relations

Vicious circles. One person is aggressive to another, the behaviour is returned and so it goes round in a circle. The object is to break the circle. Return aggression with kindness. This may sound obvious but it works.

Drink
It is easy to find out if you have a drink problem. Stop drinking for a bit and see what happens. If you are worried there are a number of things you can do. First, try to remember how you got where you are. Has stress led to a gradual increase in consumption? If so, no action on the drinking is likely to succeed unless the underlying stress is dealt with. Most 'social alcoholics' have remarkable power to regulate their intake once the problem is identified. If this is unsuccessful, you can get specialist help. Staff medical officers may be helpful, but often there is a reluctance to visit them in case you are labelled as having a problem. Agencies such as Alcoholics Anonymous are reliable and discreet.

Absenteeism
Try not to do it. Better, though, to take a day or two off than blow up completely.

Anger and irritability
Another vicious circle. Try hard not to be irritable with colleagues and nursing staff because this will lead to a withdrawal of cooperation and a worsening of the stress that led to the irritability in the first place.

Burnout
If you can see it coming, either in yourself or in colleagues, take urgent steps to decrease pressure (prioritize, delegate) and to strengthen defences (take time off, go on holiday). Don't forget that being a junior doctor is a temporary state of affairs and that, if all else fails, you can always resign and go somewhere else or do something different.

COVERING FOR COLLEAGUES/ROTAS

You will find that you are contractually obliged to cover for colleagues for short periods of absence (e.g. illness). Your contract will probably state that this should not be for prolonged or excessive periods of time. The question as to what period of time is prolonged or excessive is open. Where colleagues are absent for long periods, locums or temporary appointments should be made.

The term 'prospective cover' is used to mean the provision of cover on a predictable basis, i.e. for holidays and study leave. Your contract is likely to require you to provide this and it has advantages for the administrator:

• It is cheaper than locum cover
• It is more reliable in the sense that you are a 'known quantity'

- It means that whatever mess is made of the leave arrangements, the junior staff and not the administrators will be left to sort it out.

If you are required to cover prospectively for colleagues, this should be accounted for in your UMT payments.

If you are being underpaid or overworked or both, then the objectives for action are:

- To be reimbursed for work done
- To be paid properly for what you are doing
- To have your workload reduced.

These objectives can be reached (in order of difficulty) by:

- Asking your Consultant to intervene
- Asking the BMA to intervene (if you are a member)
- Following one of the procedures for industrial grievances.

The threat of claiming all reimbursement retrospectively at the standard UMT rate (which you are entitled to do) can have a marvellous effect on administrators. Make sure, though, that you keep a careful record of the exact time and date for each period of extra duty and, if you send it to anyone, keep a photocopy.

Where colleagues fail to pull their weight or are persistently absent, you may be able to persuade them by peer pressure to improve their performance. Failing this, you may have to go to a senior colleague to see if they can improve the situation. As a last resort, the medical staffing officer should be alerted if somebody consistently takes time off. You should not drive yourself mad by trying to do work that isn't yours and which you can't manage.

STUDY LEAVE AND HOLIDAYS

The amount of study leave and holiday due to you is usually set out in your contract. Make sure you take them. Nobody will thank you for not taking your holidays and you should find useful things to do with your study leave so that you can get trained.

House jobs are supposed to be training posts and you are entitled to find suitable courses to go on. Although medical management will try very hard not to pay you to go on courses, it has no right to do this and with the support of your Consultant, you should be able to win in most cases. The BMA will also support you if you are a member.

It is wise to give as much notice as possible about prospective holidays, because both medical and management staff may not unreasonably require that key members of staff are not away at the same time. If you have a particular date booked, you should give as much notice as possible; this may even mean identifying times before you start a post, if you know you are going to a particular rotation. A minimum of 6 weeks is usually required to be sure of time off, even if nobody else is away. Any less notice than this and the management is entitled to turn you down.

Payment in lieu of holidays is not normally available for short periods of time unless there was some special reason for not being able to take leave (such as a colleague being ill), so there is no advantage in failing to take your allotted time off. In addition, you need it and no reasonable Consultant will try and lean on you to take less than your full allowance.

GETTING YOUR NEXT JOB

Choosing the job

Which job should you go for?
Obviously this will depend on a number of factors including:

- What do you want to do?
- Why?
- Where do you want to be in 10 years' time?
- Will the job help you to achieve your long-term aims?
- What are your aims and objectives for this particular post?
- Where will you go after you have finished this job?

Where do you want to be?

- Does the job exist in a place where you would like to live?
- Is it suitable for your immediate family (wife, children), your relations (parents, grandparents), or for social recreational facilities that you particularly want or require?

If you want to work locally in your career post then it may be as well to stay in the immediate area if training is relatively short (e.g. general practice). If you want to train in a hospital specialty, there is time to move around a bit and it will certainly make your CV stronger.

Try and be in the area you want to remain in immediately before your career appointment.

How do you exercise your choice?
Once you have decided on the sort of post you want and the area in which you would like to work, you should:

- Identify which posts will come up during the time when you need a job.
- Show interest before the job is advertised. This will make the people who are making the appointment realize that you are serious.
- When an appropriate post is advertised try to go and see the job before shortlisting takes place. It is probably not necessary or even desirable to try and see all the

Consultants at this stage, but an early interest expressed
and a visit to the centre will help you to get a feel for what
is required and, therefore, to prepare your CV accordingly.

Getting on the shortlist

The keys to this both have the initials CV:

- Crawling Vigourously
- Curriculum Vitae.

Crawling vigourously

It is sometimes not thought to be desirable or necessary to see
individual Consultants about jobs in advance, although if they
are within your own hospital or immediate area, this is clearly
at least a courtesy, if not a necessity. The degree of ingratiation
that can be managed will vary from applicant to applicant.

The degree and means of ingratiation should also be tailored
to each Consultant. General rules are:

- Try to make an appointment to see everyone on the
  shortlisting committee.
- If you succeed, turn up on time and ask urbane questions.
- Be keen but not manic.
- Explain *why* you want the job, if you can.
- (Try and be related to as many members of the committee
  as possible!)

Curriculum vitae

This should be produced to a very high standard, and either
typed well or better still produced on a word processor with
laser printing. Something poorly prepared, poorly typed, poorly
arranged or on poor quality paper will go straight into the bin.

In areas where you are not known, the Committee will only
have your CV to go on in deciding who to shortlist and you
must therefore make a strong claim.

There are no hard and fast rules for the way in which a CV
is constructed, but there is a basic outline.

Personal and administrative details   Under this heading you
should include your:

- Name
- Home address
- Home telephone number
- Hospital address
- Hospital telephone number
- Date of birth/age
- Nationality
- Marital status
- GMC registration number/type.

Education   Include (with dates) your:

- School
- University and medical school qualifications

- Present post
- Academic awards, grants
- Distinctions and scholarships.

Posts Give a chronological summary of the posts you have held with:

- Dates
- Title of the posts
- Specialty
- Consultants' names and work address (the name of the hospital).

A summary of professional experience

- Details of your day-to-day duties
- Clinics, procedures you have learnt to do
- Procedures you have done under supervision
- Procedures you have experience of (particularly if specialized).

Teaching experience Include:

- On-ward teaching of medical students
- Lectures or seminars
- Journal clubs, presentations to hospital clinical meetings.

Management experience This is worth mentioning because it is a heading that some people may be looking out for. As a House Officer you may have experience of:

- Managing the day-to-day running of the medical side of the ward
- Co-ordination of various services
- Social/sporting posts when an undergraduate.

Research Include:

- Research in progress if you are involved in any projects
- Research you have already completed (recently or as a student or during a previous degree).

Publications Normally listed in the order:

- Books
- Book chapters
- Original papers
- Abstracts.

Presentations

- Invitations
- Presentations to learned societies.

Non-medical interests Limited to two or three at the very most, but can be included:

- To show some breadth of interests outside medicine
- To give something to ask you about at interview.

Referees They must be informed, both that you are seeking a job and that you have named them as a referee. This is best done by seeking their advice before you apply, rather than presenting them with this fact as a *fait accomplis*. Give the address where they will actually see the letter requesting a reference (home, private rooms).

It is quite common for application forms to be sent out to be filled-in for jobs. These also need to be prepared in a neat way and to be accurate. Don't try and cram a lot of detail into too small a space. As these forms are primarily for administrative purposes, it is perfectly OK to write in the appropriate space, 'Please see attached curriculum vitae', which you should always send in any case.

Every curriculum vitae, application form and application should be accompanied by a handwritten letter on headed paper from your present employment. This should:

- Formally express your intention to apply for the job
- Make note of the enclosed application forms and CV
- State your career objectives and intent (though many prefer to have a paragraph or two on this within the CV).

Getting the job

Before the interview

Once shortlisted you *must* see all persons involved in appointing the post on the Consultant's staff. This may mean several visits and can be quite onerous, but is absolutely essential. You will not be appointed by people who haven't met you before. (If the Consultant's secretary says that the Consultant is not seeing anybody, you can breathe a sigh of relief; otherwise you *must* visit.)

Prepare questions to ask. The purpose of your visit is supposed not to be to ingratiate yourself, but to assess the post. Ask about training, research or any other specific intelligent question you can come up with. Questions about time off, holidays and industrial relations rarely go down well.

Go over your CV to identify strengths and weaknesses and be prepared to talk on any subject contained therein.

The interview

- Be on time
- Be smartly dressed (suit or equivalent – this is no time for a fashion statement)
- Be ready to discuss:
  - Your education
  - Jobs you have done
  - Why you want this job
  - Your choice of career (you may be questioned vigourously on this)
  - What will happen in your chosen specialty in your professional lifetime

- Where you see yourself in 2, 5, 10 years time (not in a mirror!)
- The implications of any move on your family
- Outside interests
- (Anything else at all that any nosy beggar fancies asking you!)

- Be up to date with what is happening in the medical world
- Always be polite
- Don't get rattled (defensive, aggressive, flippant)
- Never criticize (the Committee may actually *like* your old boss who is an absolute swine)
- Agree to take the job if offered (no ifs or buts).

The final question at the interview is, 'Have you any questions?' The answer is *always* no. You should have asked them before interview – remember?

Once you have got the job

Get a contract of employment before you resign any existing post. Check that the UMTs correlate with the rota and that the standard terms and conditions exist.

If you have time it may be worth inspecting the accommodation to make sure it is of sufficient standard, although there may not be very much you can do about it.

Telephone the incumbent doctors and ask about rotas and the various ins and outs of the job. It is no good trying to find out more about the job once you have arrived, because all the people who know the most about it will have moved on.

If you must take holiday near the beginning of the job, be sure to write and give as much notice as possible, preferably with reasons as to why the holiday must be taken at this time.

14

Pathology services

257

Labelling of samples

- Label each specimen with the patient's name and hospital number.
- A completed and legible request form must accompany each specimen. This must bear the patient's full name (surname and forename), sex, age, ward and hospital number, the name of the Consultant and name and bleep of the requesting doctor. The type of specimen and investigation required should be given, as well as the time and date when the specimen was collected. Relevant clinical details of current, recent or proposed treatment should also be noted as these may affect the way in which the specimen is processed and the interpretation of the results.
- High-risk specimens should be clearly labelled 'Biohazard' and the precise hazard given (see below).

Transport of samples

Fixative, special containers and transport boxes, if required, are obtainable from the laboratory on request. Ensure that the tops of bottles, etc. are securely fastened to prevent leakage. Each specimen should be enclosed in a suitably sized, sealed plastic bag and accompanied by its own request form.

Potentially infectious samples

Specimens from patients with certain infectious diseases are a potential hazard to those handling them. The usual policy is to label *both* specimen and request form with a biohazard sticker. The nature of the hazard should be indicated in the clinical details. Specimens from the following groups should be so labelled:

- Known HBsAg carriers
- Suspected cases of acute hepatitis, until cleared by the responsible clinician
- Patients known to be HIV positive, or in a high-risk group
  - Homosexual and bisexual men
  - Intravenous drug abusers
  - Haemophiliacs and others who may have received contaminated blood products in the management of disease
  - Those who have recently lived or worked in Central and Southern Africa
  - The sexual partners and infant children of the above groups
- Known or strongly suspected cases of typhoid or paratyphoid fever until cleared by a Microbiologist
- Known or strongly suspected cases of tuberculosis including proven cases whilst on anti-tuberculosis therapy
- Other cases as requested by the Control of Infection Officer or Microbiologist.

Use a separate plastic bag marked with the biohazard symbol. Place the sample in the bag and seal by removing the paper strip and folding the flap into the adhesive band. Roll the bag up and place it into a normal specimen bag.

Delays may be experienced in the processing of samples and some investigations may not be performed owing to the hazard represented to laboratory personnel. Some departments may restrict work done on certain samples.

If you have a patient within a risk group and are in doubt about the feasibility of a test, contact the laboratory concerned to discuss the request.

Urgent and out-of-hours requests

If the result of a test is urgent, phone the laboratory first – it is not sufficient simply to label the sample 'urgent'. Also, remember it is your responsibility to see the sample arrives in the laboratory.

Out-of-hours requests must also be preceded by a telephone call to the laboratory concerned. These tests are expensive and must be restricted to those important for the *immediate* management of a patient, i.e. if further clinical action can only proceed with the result of the test.

Non-urgent samples sent to the laboratory out of hours will not be processed until the following morning.

HAEMATOLOGY

The investigations carried out by the Haematology laboratory are listed in Table 14.1

A Consultant must approve the following tests:

- Red cell and plasma volume
- Red cell survival
- Osmotic fragility
- Tests for unstable haemoglobin
- Detailed studies to investigate haemolytic anaemia.

THE BLOOD TRANSFUSION LABORATORY

This is used for the grouping and cross-matching of blood.

> **Remember**
>
> Blood transfusion is the same as organ transplantation and is the most frequently performed transplant procedure. As much care must be taken with cross-matching as is taken with tissue typing for transplantation.

Table 14.1
Haematology tests

Investigation	Volume (ml)	Container	Comments
FBC (WCC, RCC, Hb, PCV, MCV, MCHC and inspection of film)	4	Sequestrene (EDTA)	
Haemoglobin electrophoresis + quantification of A2	4	Sequestrene (EDTA)	
Prothrombin time	2 (exactly)	Citrate; mauve label (Do *not* use ESR citrate tube)	
ESR	2 (exactly)	ESR citrate tube with peforated cap	
Serum B12	10	Plain bottle	
Prothrombin time, activated partial thromboplastin time (aPTT), thrombin time	4.5 (exactly)	Citrate; mauve label (Do *not* use ESR citrate tube)	NB: Under- and over-filled bottles cannot be accepted for coagulation studies as results are inaccurate. Contact the laboratory before taking samples from polycythaemic patients

Table 14.1 *(contd)*
Haematology tests

Investigation	Volume (ml)	Container	Comments
Fibrin/fibrinogen degradation products (FDP)	2 (exactly)	Special bottle obtained from laboratory	Ensure specimen is sent whenever DIC is suspected
Capillary prothrombin time			Send patient to laboratory by arrangement
Platelet aggregation studies	9	Citrate; mauve label (Do *not* use ESR bottle)	
Glucose-6-phosphate dehydrogenase deficiency	4	Sequestrene (EDTA)	
Urinary haemosiderin	10 (urine)	Plain bottle	Early morning specimen
Haptoglobin	5	Plain bottle	
Plasma haemoglobin	4	Sequestrene (EDTA)	
Ferritin	5	Plain bottle	
Group, screen for antibodies and retain serum	10	Plain bottle	This sample can be used for cross-matching for 1 week after receipt

Table 14.1 (*contd*)
Haematology tests

Investigation	Volume (ml)	Container	Comments
Cross-match (for each 6 units)	10	Plain bottle	A minimum of 24 h and preferably 48 h is required for non-urgent transfusion
Direct antiglobulin test	4	Sequestrene (EDTA)	
Malaria parasites	4	Sequestrene (EDTA)	Can be done on same sample as FBC but full clinical details are required
Cold agglutinins			Consult the blood transfusion laboratory in advance as a warm specimen is required

The minimum labelling requirements for transfusion request forms are:

- Surname and forename; always use the same names and spell them correctly
- Date of birth
- Case number or A & E number.

If you delegate the job of venesection for transfusion specimens to another person, make sure he/she understands the importance of careful patient identification.

Also, indicate the diagnosis or surgical procedure for each patient.

Type of specimen

- Clotted blood – for grouping and cross-matching
- EDTA (sequestrene) blood for a direct antiglobulin test.

Notice required for provision of blood

A full working day is usually required for the safe provision of blood unless the patient's blood has already been grouped and screened for irregular antibodies from the outpatient clinic. It is frequently impossible to provide compatible blood at short notice for patients with irregular antibodies.

Recall of blood

Any units that are unused within 24 h of the time for which they were requested will be cross-matched for another patient. If you want to delay a transfusion, let the laboratory know in good time.

Transfusion of blood

Identification checks at this stage are critical. The giving of blood should be regarded in the same way as the giving of dangerous drugs. A check must be carried out by two persons, at least one of whom must be a doctor, state registered nurse, state certified midwife or state enrolled nurse. Their signature should be recorded on the blood transfusion form. Check:

- Number on the unit and on the form correspond
- ABO and Rh group correspond on unit and form
- Unit against form for patient's name, forename, hospital number and the ward
- Name and number of unit and form against identification details, either on the patient's bracelet or in the patient's notes.

Haematological normal values:

Hb	13.5–18 g/dl
WBC	$4–11 \times 10^9$/l
PLT	$150–400 \times 10^9$/l
Sodium	135–145 mmol/l
Potassium	3.6–5.0 mmol/l
Bicarbonate	22–30 mmol/l
Urea	1.7–7.1 mmol/l
Creatinine	55–125 µmol/l
Glucose	3.5–7.0 mmol/l
Bilirubin	0–22 µmol/l
Alkaline phosphatase	38–126 U/l
Albumin	35–50 g/l
Calcium	2.2–2.55 mmol/l
Amylase	0–110 U/l

CYTOLOGY/CYTOGENETICS

The following information may not cover all eventualities, and when any doubt exists as to the optimum way in which a sample should be collected and sent to the laboratory, telephone the laboratory for instructions *before the specimen is obtained*.

Effusions

A minimum of 100 ml of fluid should be sent to the laboratory in a sterile container. If it has a tendency to clot, 20 ml of 3.8 M sodium citrate solution should be added and gently mixed. It is *essential* to state clearly when an anticoagulant has been added.

Urine

A minimum of 20 ml of voided urine should be sent. A catheter or mid-stream specimen is *not* satisfactory for cytological investigation. If the only specimen available is a catheter one, this must be clearly stated on the request form.

Urine should be collected into a sterile container and sent to the laboratory immediately whilst fresh. Cell morphology deteriorates rapidly in voided urine and specimens more than a few hours old may be unsatisfactory for a reliable cytological assessment.

Respiratory tract specimens

Sputum Early morning specimens should be sent fresh to the laboratory and collected on 3 consecutive days. Check the quantity is adequate and sputum is not contaminated with food, saliva, tobacco or toothpaste. A specimen after physiotherapy, or postural drainage, is very useful.

Bronchial aspirate   Can be useful if suction is prolonged for 1 min and the bronchoscope is directed towards the site of the lesion. The aspirate should be collected into a sterile container and sent immediately to the laboratory. Trap specimens can be sent in the same way.

Bronchial brush/touch preparation   Smears made from bronchial brushings/biopsies should be spread evenly and quickly on clearly labelled, clean glass slides and immersed immediately in 95% alcohol. Avoid any air drying, since this will affect cell preservation and impair staining and evaluation.

Bronchoalveolar lavages/induced sputum   These specimens should be taken into sterile containers and sent immediately to the laboratory.

Nipple discharge

The discharge should be smeared onto a slide and fixed immediately whilst wet. Suitable fixatives are Spraycyte, Cytofix or 95% industrial methylated spirit.

Aspirates

Breast cysts   These should be expressed into a sterile container. Fixative is not necessary, but can be used (50% normal saline and 50% alcohol fixative can be obtained from the Cytology laboratory on request). If fixative is added, this *must* be clearly stated, since laboratory processing will be different and the wrong procedure may render the specimen unsatisfactory.

Solid tumour   Appropriate for lymph nodes and solid tumours of breast. Using a No. 1 needle and syringe, aspirate the tumour and express material onto a slide. Spread as for a blood film and fix *immediately* in a jar of 95% alcohol or Spraycyte. If the amount of material aspirated is small, wash out the syringe with 3 ml of a fixative solution made up of equal parts of normal saline and 95% alcohol.

Air-dried smears may be required for Romanowsky stains or special procedures. It is essential that any such smears are spread thinly and dried quickly.

Smear preparation and staining in the laboratory is quite different so it is essential that air-dried and wet-fixed smears are clearly labelled. The wrong procedure will render the specimens unsatisfactory for cytological assessment.

Fine needle   A member of the laboratory staff will always come to the clinic to prepare smears from fine-needle aspirate (FNA). If an immediate assessment is needed, e.g. in ultrasound or X-ray, an appointment should be made with the cytology laboratory for a pathologist to be present at the time of the FNA.

CSF and joint   Send as much of the specimen as can be spared to the cytology laboratory, unfixed. Do *not* freeze. If there is unavoidable delay in sending a fresh specimen to the laboratory, it should be stored at 4°C.

> **Remember**
>
> As a general rule, unfixed specimens >12 h old, which have not been refrigerated, are unsuitable for reliable cytological assessment.

Scrapes from skin or oral lesions

Scrapings should be spread onto a slide and fixed immediately whilst wet with Cytofix, Spraycyte or 95% industrial methylated spirit. This method is useful for detecting basal cell carcinoma. Ambulant patients can usually be referred to the cytology department, where the specimen will be taken and a diagnosis made on the spot. Make appointments in advance.

BIOCHEMISTRY

Indications for biochemical tests

Electrolytes

- Myocardial infarction
- Abnormal cardiac rhythms with/without myocardial infarction
- Chest infection (only where blood gases are also indicated)
- Acute presentation of diabetes
- Known or suspected abnormalities of renal function
- Clouding of consciousness where there are no obvious gross CNS signs
- Signicant hypovolaemia, e.g.:
  - Multiple injuries
  - Severe diarrhoea and vomiting
  - Intestinal obstruction
  - Burns: <20% in adults; >10% in children, or where burns are in critical areas (hands, face and perineum)
  - Patients who are on drugs that may affect electrolyte balance, or drugs that are affected by abnormalities of electrolytes
  - Patients who are on TPN.

Urea/creatinine

- Suspected renal failure
- Unexplained gross electrolyte abnormalities
- Significant hypovolaemia (as above)
- Clouding of consciousness where there are no obvious gross CNS signs
- Acute retention of urine
- Unexplained pericarditis.

Glucose

- Acute presentation of diabetes
- Epilepsy*
- Insulin coma*
- Drug overdose*
- Diabetic patients presenting with other pathology*.
  (*Only to confirm doubtful BM Stix readings.)

Amylase

- Abdominal pain/trauma with a high index of suspicion of pancreatitis.

Blood gases

- Respiratory problems where there is:
  - Asthma
  - Cyanosis
  - Clouding of consciousness
  - Apparent need of artificial ventilation
  - Chest injures/flail chest
  - Pulmonary/fat embolism/respiratory distress syndrome
  - A disease (or suspicion of a disease) that may cause clinically unrecognized hypoxia (e.g. acute pancreatitis)
  - Postcardiac arrest
  - Acute presentation of diabetes.

Calcium

- Post-parathyroidectomy/thyroidectomy
- Clinical signs and symptoms of tetany in patients who are not hyperventilating
- Clinical symptoms/signs suggestive of hypercalcaemia
- Acute pancreatitis.

Biochemical samples left unseparated overnight will be unsuitable for the analysis of potassium, phosphate and certain enzymes.

Blood and urine tests (Tables 14.2 and 14.3)

It is exremely difficult to define reference ranges as these are influenced by a large number of variables: sex, age, race, time of day, etc. The adult reference ranges given in Tables 14.2 and 14.3 are only a guide. Laboratory advice should be sought in case of difficulty, and to confirm the reference ranges at your hospital.

Faecal specimens

Faecal fat excretion   A 3-day collection is the minimum period for which a reliable result may be obtained. If a patient has infrequent motions and mild malabsorption, a 5-day collection is recommended. It is important that this type of patient has an adequate fat intake (>100 g/day), as normal faecal fat results

Table 14.2
Biochemical blood tests

Investigation	Container	Minimum volume (ml)	Reference range
Aldosterone	Heparinized	5	
Antitrypsin	Plain	5	1.0–2.2 g/l
Amylase	Plain	5	<1000 U/l
Bicarbonate (T/CO$_2$)	Heparinized venous blood	5	24–30 mmol/l
(brought to lab in a sealed syringe)			
Bilirubin	Heparinized	5	5–17 µmol/l
Caeruloplasmin	Plain	5	0.2–0.6 g/l
Calcium	Heparinized	5	2.12–2.55 mmol/l
Cholesterol	Plain	10	<5.2 mmol/l – desirable 5.2–6.5 mmol/l – borderline >6.5 mmol/l – high
HDL-cholesterol	Plain		>0.9 mmol/l
Chloride	Heparinized	5	95–105 mmol/l
Cortisol	Heparinized	5	170–600 nmol/l
Copper	Plain	5	11–20 µmol/l
Creatinine kinase	Heparinized	5	24–190 U/l
Creatinine	Heparinized	5	60–125 µmol/l
Dehydrogenases (LDH)	Heparinized	5	150–450 U/l
Electrolytes	Heparinized	5	
Na$^+$			135–145 mmol/l
K$^+$			3.5–5.0 mmol/l
Fibrinogen	Sodium citrate	5	2–4.5 g/l
FSH	Plain	5	
Gases (arrange by telephone)	Heparinized arterial blood	5	
pH			7.35–7.45
pCO$_2$			35–45 mmHg
pO$_2$			90–110 mmHg
Actual bicarbonate			22–27 mmol/l
Base excess			−3 to +3 mmol/l
Glucose (and for CSF)	Fluoride oxalate	4	Fasting 3–5 mmol/l
Gamma glutamyl transferase	Heparinized	5	Male <50 U/l Female <32 U/l
HBAI	EDTA	5	<8% total
Immunoglobulins	Plain	5	IgG 6–17 g/l IgA 0.7–3.5 g/l IgM 0.5–2.5 g/l

Table 14.2 (*contd*)
Biochemical blood tests

Investigation	Container	Minimum volume (ml)	Reference range
Iron	Plain	10	9–29 µmol/l
LH	Plain	5	
Lithium	Plain	5	0.6–1.2 mmol/l
Liver function tests	Heparinized	5	
Bilirubin			5–17 µmol/l
Alkaline phosphatase (adults)			30–130 U/l
Aspartate transaminase			7–40 U/l
Total protein			60–80 g/l
Albumin			35–51 g/l
Magnesium	Plain	5	0.65–1.0 mmol/l
Osmolality	Heparinized	5	280–295 mmol/kg
Phosphatases			
Alkaline	Heparinized	5	30–130 U/l
Acid			
– Total	Plain	5	<7 U/l
– Prostatic			<4 U/l
Phosphate	Heparinized	10	0.8–1.4 mmol/l
Progesterone	Plain	2	
Prolactin	Plain	2	<520 U/l
Protein electrophoresis	Plain	5	
Salicylates	Plain	10	
Testosterone	Plain	5	
Thyroid function tests:	Plain	5	
Thyroxine			50–150 nmol/l
TSH			0.5–6.5 mU/l
Free T3			2.9–8.9 pmol/l
Transferrin	Plain	10	2.0–4.0 g/l
Triglyceride (fasting)	Plain	10	<2.1 mmol/l
Urea	Heparinized	5	2.5–6.6 mmol/l
Urate	Heparinized	5	0.15–0.45 mmol/l
Zinc	Plain	10	11–24 µmol/l

**Table 14.3
Biochemical urine tests**

Investigation	Container	Minimum quantity	Reference range
Amino acids	Universal	EMU 20 ml (fresh)	Qualitative
Bilirubin and urobilinogen	Universal	20 ml Random	Qualitative
Calcium	Acidified (HCl)[†]	24 h	2.5–10.0 mmol/24 h
Copper	Plain (acid washed)	24 h	0.25–0.8 µmol/24 h
Cortisol	Plain	24 h	20–300 nmol/24 h
Creatinine*	Plain	24 h	9–17 mmol/24 h
Electrolytes	Plain	24 h	
Sodium			110–240 mmol/24 h
Potassium			35–100 mmol/24 h
Urea			250–580 mmol/24 h
5HIAA	Acidified (acetic acid)[†]	24 h	36–52 µmol/24 h
HMMA (VMA)	Acidified (HCL)[†]	24 h	<40 µmol/24 h
Osmolality	Universal	20 ml	Very variable Random
Oxalate	Acidified (HCl)[†]	24 h	<40 mg/24 h
Phosphate	Plain	24 h	16–48 mmol/24 h
Porphyrins and porphobilinogen	Universal	EMU 20 ml (fresh)	Qualitative
Protein	Plain	24 h	<0.1 g/24 h
Bence–Jones	Universal	EMU 20 ml	
Uric acid	Plain	24 h	3–12 mmol/24 h

* Send accompanying blood sample for clearance.
[†] Acidified containers available from diagnostic chemical pathology.

may be obtained in patients with steatorrhoea on a low fat intake. It should be appreciated that this test is unpleasant to perform and labour intensive.

Specimens are collected in tins, which may be obtained from the laboratory. These tins should not be filled more than half-way, otherwise the analysis cannot be carried out. Large containers for patients passing bulky stools may be obtained on request.

This analysis should not be performed if the patient suffers from diarrhoea or is taking laxatives.

MICROBIOLOGY

- All blood cultures should be sent immediately to the appropriate bacteriology department for incubation at 37°C.
- Sputum samples received in the laboratory > 12 h after being taken, and salivary specimens, are not cultured for respiratory pathogens other than tuberculosis.
- Unless inpatient urine specimens are clearly unrepeatable, e.g. because treatment is about to be started, they will not be processed if received > 12 h after being taken.

Antibiotic assays

Assays of *gentamicin*, *netilmicin* and *vancomycin* can be performed on a routine basis.

- Trough level: take blood immediately before the dose
- Peak level: (i.m./i.v.) take blood 30 min after the dose.

Results of levels taken at a different interval can be validly interpreted, so include the time of dose and level on the request form.

Blood should be collected in a plain tube (at least 2 ml blood needed) or, in the case of SCBU patients, in small plastic containers (minimum sample 100 µl).

In the case of weekend requests it is helpful to contact the laboratory with advance warning on Friday.

Other assays are not performed routinely. These must be discussed with a member of the medical staff and, if required, may necessitate considerable forward planning.

The investigations available from the Microbiology Department are listed in Table 14.4.

Serology

All tests (Table 14.5) require about 5–10 ml of clotted blood. Tests sent to reference laboratories:

- Amoebic FAT/CFT
- Antistreptolysin
- Hydatid CFT
- Toxocara.

Tuberculosis

When sputum and urine samples are investigated for TB, three pooled specimens are generally examined together and the samples are not processed until the set of three is complete.

Table 14.4
Microbiology investigations

Specimen	Investigation	Container/ swab	Average time for report
Antral w/out	Micro/culture	Universal	48 h
BAL	Micro/culture	Sterilin mucus trap	48 h/5 days
	TB culture	Sterilin mucus trap	8 weeks
Blood	Antibiotic assay	Plain blood tube	
	Routine culture	Blood culture set	48 h/7 days
	Brucella culture	Blood culture set	3 weeks
	Leptospira culture		
	Serology	Plain blood tube	
CSF	Micro/culture	Universal	24 h/48 h
	Syphilis serology	Universal	24 h
Ear swab	Micro/culture	ENT swab*	48 h
Eye swab	Micro/culture	Transwab*	48 h
	Conjunctival scrape	Transwab*	48 h
	Chlamydia IF	Microtrak slide	Same day
Faeces	Culture	60 ml container	48–72 h
	Parasitology	60 ml container	1–4 days
	Clostridium difficile	60 ml container	2–5 days
Joint fluid	Micro/culture	Universal	48 h
	GC culture	Universal	72 h
	TB culture	Universal	8 weeks
Nose swab	Culture	Transwab*	24 h
Pernasal	Bordetella culture	Pernasal swab*	5 days
PD fluid	Micro/culture	Universal	48 h
Pus	Micro/culture	Universal	48 h
	TB culture	Universal	8 weeks
SCBU screen	Culture	answab*	48–72 h
Skin swab	Micro/culture	answab*	48 h

Table 14.4 (contd)
Microbiology investigations

Sputum	Micro/culture	60 ml container	24–48 h
	TB culture	60 ml container	8 weeks
	Eosinophils	60 ml container	24 h
Throat swab	Culture	Transwab*	24 h
Tissue	Micro/culture	60 ml container	48–72 h
	TB culture	60 ml container	8 weeks
Urine			
MSU/CSU	Micro/culture	Universal	24 h
EMU	TB culture	Honey pot	8 weeks
Terminal EMU	Schistosomes	Universal	Same day
Vaginal/ cervical/ urethral	Micro/culture (includes GC, Candida, TV)	Transwab*	48 h
Wound swab	Micro/culture	Transwab*	48 h

* Do not send dry swabs for investigation

Table 14.5
Serology tests

Test	Average time for report	Comment
Brucella agglutination	2–4 days	Confirmation by reference lab
Legionella RMAT	1–2 days	Usually done once a week
Paul-Bunnell	1–2 days	Usually unneccessary
Syphilis VDRL/TPHA/FTA	24 h	
Toxoplasma	1–2 days	Confirmation by reference lab
Widal	1–2 days	Seldom indicated

If you require immediate microscopy, contact the laboratory to request this investigation. The result will then be phoned to you. If a set of specimens is incomplete, a reminder is sent out. Unless further specimens are received or the laboratory is contacted to request the processing of the incomplete set, the samples received will be discarded.

Cultures are incubated for up to 8 weeks (12 weeks in the case of CSF) before being discarded as negative.

VIROLOGY

The tests available from the Virology Department are listed in Table 14.6.

To maximize the chances of isolating virus it is necessary that the specimen reaches the laboratory as soon as possible. The specimens should be sent on ice. If there is any delay in transporting specimens, they should be kept at $+4°C$. Failure to observe this precaution will increase viral death and increase the growth of contaminating bacteria and fungi.

Viruses are for the most part intracellular parasites. It is most important to remember this, especially when taking throat

Table 14.6
Virology investigations

Investigation	Container
Serology:	
HIV antibody and antigen tests	10 ml of i.v. blood into plain tube
Hepatitis B surface antigen	
Hepatitis B antibodies	
Hepatitis A antibodies	
Rubella antibodies	
Complement fixation tests	
Other viral serology tests	
Isolation of virus from:	
Blood	10 ml of i.v. blood into plain tube with 'preservative-free' heparin (not lithium), 10 U heparin/ml of blood
Urine	MSU into 30 ml universal container (undiluted)
Stool	60 ml container
CSF and vesicle fluid	As much as can be obtained into 30 ml universal container (undiluted)
Bronchial alveolar lavage	Mucus extractor
Needle biopsy	Virus transport medium
Swabs	Virus transport medium
Nasopharyngeal aspirate	Sterilin mucus trap

swabs and nasopharyngeal aspirates. It is a waste of time to process these specimens unless they contain cellular material. The soft palate on either side of the uvula is a good place for swabbing the throat.

IMMUNOLOGY

Autoantibodies

10 ml of clotted blood is needed for the following investigations:

- Antinuclear factor (ANF)
- DNA binding (double-sranded) (DNAB)
- Extractable nuclear antigen (ENA)
- Antimitochondrial antibody
- Smooth muscle antibody
- Gastric parietal cell antibody
- Thyroid antibodies
  - Microsomal antibody
  - Thyroglobulin antibody
- Rheumatoid factors
  - Latex
  - RAHA.

Other specific autoantibodies, e.g. anti-islet cell antibodies, are performed at regional centres, but should be sent to Microbiology/Biochemistry (depending upon local facilities), where they will be redirected.

Complement

For complement analysis, 5 ml of blood in EDTA (an 'FBC' bottle) is required.

- Total haemolytic complement
- C3
- C4
- C3d (complement activation product)
- C1 esterase inhibitor.

C-reactive protein

- Quantative
- Latex (semi-quantative, urgent samples only, same day result). This can be performed on small quantities of blood, i.e. 0.5 ml.

Total and specific IgE levels (Prist and Rast)

10 ml of clotted blood is needed. Specify which RASTs are required – a list of currently available allergens can be obtained from the Biochemistry/Microbiology Departments of your hospital.

Cryoglobulins

Blood needs to be taken into a prewarmed syringe and bottle and transported to the laboratory at 37°C.

APPENDIX

Patients often don't know their weight in kilograms:

Stones	Kilograms (kg)
1	6.4
2	12.7
5	31.8
6	38.2
7	44.5
8	50.9
9	57.3
10	63.6
11	70.0
12	76.4
13	82.7
14	89.1
15	95.5
16	101.8
17	108.2
18	114.5
19	120.9
20	127.2

Index

F

G

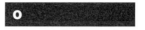

USEFUL TELEPHONE AND BLEEP NUMBERS

Consultant _____

Consultant _____

Consultant _____

Consultant _____

Consultant _____

Consultant _____

Senior Registrar _____

Registrar _____

SHO _____

Anaesthetist _____

Anaesthetist _____

Anaesthetist _____

Anaesthetist _____

Accident & Emergency _____

Administrator _____

Biochemistry _____

Blood Transfusion Service _____

Cardiology _____

Chest Physician _____

Cytology _____

Dentist _____

Dermatology _____

ENT _____

Gastroenterology _____

Gynaecology _____

Haematology _____

Immunology _____

Microbiology _____

Neurology _____

Nursing Officer _____

Paediatrics _____

Pathology _____